This book is one of the titles in the series of
Wolfe Medical Atlases, a series which brings
together probably the world's largest systematic
published collection of diagnostic colour
photographs.
For a full list of Atlases in the series, plus
forthcoming titles and details of our surgical,
dental and veterinary Atlases, please write to
Wolfe Medical Publications Limited,
3–5 Conway Street,
London W1P 6HE

Series Editor: G. Barry Carruthers, MD(London)

Copyright © R. Hall, D. Evered, R. Greene, 1979
Published by Wolfe Medical Publications Ltd, 1979
Printed by Smeets-Weert, Holland
ISBN 0 7234 0411 9

Introduction

Our objective in compiling this atlas was to illustrate the clinical features of endocrine disorders.

Endocrinology is a specialty with a large but variable visual content. Some topics such as thyroid and pituitary diseases are largely visual, whereas others, including aldosteronism and phaeochromocytoma, have a very small visual content. We have therefore attempted to overcome this problem by introducing outline diagrams listing the clinical features of the endocrine disorders.

We have been deliberately selective in the choice of text and illustration. This atlas should therefore be used alongside a standard textbook of endocrinology.

R. Hall
D. Evered
R. Greene

Acknowledgements

The authors gratefully acknowledge the generosity of their many colleagues listed below who have allowed them to reproduce slides from their collections.

Dr J. Anderson

Dr C. N. Armstrong

Dr D. Bates

Sir Richard Bayliss

Professor G. M. Besser

Dr S. R. Bloom

Dr N. E. F. Cartlidge

Dr F. Clark

Dr C. Cooper

Professor A. Crombie

Mr D. Dawes

Mr J. R. G. Edwards

Dr J. E. Gray

Dr P. Hacking

Dr J. Haggith

Dr M. Hall

Dr G. Holti

Dr P. Hudgson

Professor J. H. Hutchinson

Dr F. A. Ive

Dr O. James

Professor I. D. A. Johnston

Dr G. F. Joplin

Dr C. R. Kanagasundaram

Dr P. A. Kendall-Taylor

Professor D. N. S. Kerr

Dr I. Lavelle

Dr J. Marks

Dr D. R. L. Newton

Dr J. P. Owen

Dr J. L. H. O'Riordan

Dr J. M. Parkin

Dr C. R. Paterson

Dr W. Price

Professor D. A. Shaw

Mr D. Tacchi

Dr J. A. Thomson

Dr A. P. Warin

Dr C. K. Warrick

Dr L. Watson

Dr G. C. Weir

Dr R. Wilkinson

Professor V. Wright

We also wish to thank Hamblin (Instruments) Limited* for allowing us to use their Scotoma charts on page 59.

*31 New Cavendish Street, London W1M 7RL.

Contents

1: Hypothalamus and pituitary

Introduction

The anterior pituitary secretes seven separate protein and polypeptide hormones. The function of the anterior pituitary is controlled by the hypothalamus, which secretes a number of regulatory factors (releasing or inhibiting hormones) (1).

1

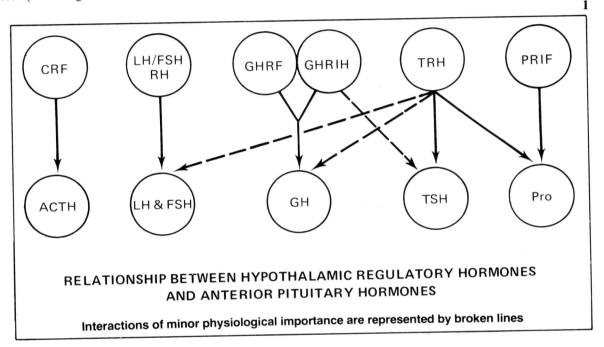

RELATIONSHIP BETWEEN HYPOTHALAMIC REGULATORY HORMONES
AND ANTERIOR PITUITARY HORMONES

Interactions of minor physiological importance are represented by broken lines

Key to Figure 1

Hypothalamic hormones

Corticotrophin-releasing factor (CRF)

Luteinising hormone/follicle-stimulating hormone-releasing hormone (LH/FSH – RH) }

Growth hormone-releasing factor (GHRF)
Growth hormone-release inhibiting hormone (GHRIH) }

Thyrotrophin-releasing hormone (TRH)

Prolactin-release inhibiting factor (PRIF)

Pituitary hormones

Corticotrophin (ACTH)

{Luteinising hormone (LH)
Follicle-stimulating hormone (FSH)

Growth hormone (GH)

Thyrotrophin (TSH)

Prolactin (Pro)

The regulatory hormones pass from the hypothalamus to the area of the median eminence by axonal flow, where they are stored and subsequently released into the capillaries of the hypothalamo-hypophysial portal system to pass to the anterior pituitary (**2**).

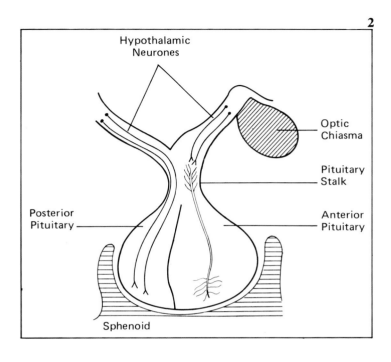

The hypothalamus plays an important role in integrating and co-ordinating pituitary function, thermostasis, water, mineral and calorie balance and sexual activity. Hypothalamic functions are modified by many environmental stimuli (physical, psychological and biochemical) and the individual releasing hormones play a part in regulating pituitary function (**3**).

The posterior pituitary is not a discrete endocrine gland but merely the distal part of an endocrine neurosecretory system, which also includes various hypothalamic areas. The antidiuretic hormone (ADH) is secreted by the hypothalamus and passes down the neurohypophysial tract linked with neurophysin to be secreted into the general circulation (**2**).

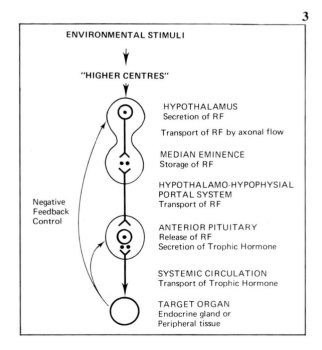

Clinical features of hypothalamic and pituitary disease

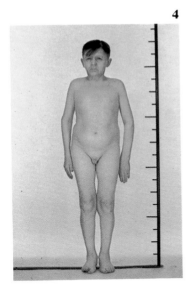

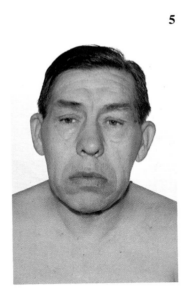

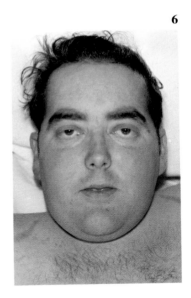

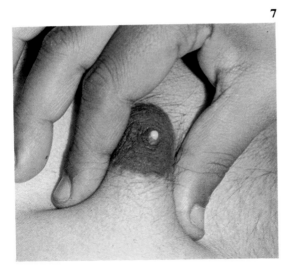

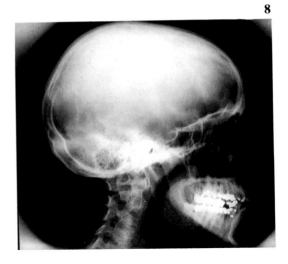

The six common clinical presentations of hypothalamic pituitary disease are as follows:

1 Partial or complete pituitary failure (**4**)

2 Acromegaly (or gigantism) (**5**)

3 Cushing's syndrome (**6**)

4 Galactorrhoea (**7**)

5 Diabetes insipidus

6 Pituitary tumour – which may be asymptomatic, or associated with any of the endocrine problems listed above or the cause of pressure effects on adjacent structures (**8**).

Pituitary failure

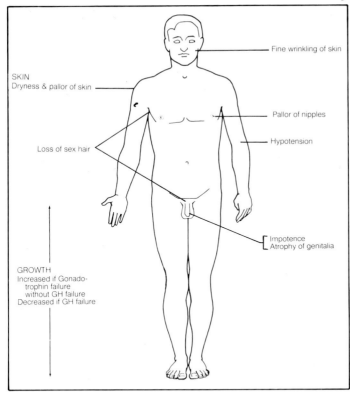

Pituitary failure commonly results from an adenoma, infarction or trauma (and occasionally from a secondary neoplasm, chronic infection, granuloma or lipoidosis). The major clinical features are shown in **9** and **10**.

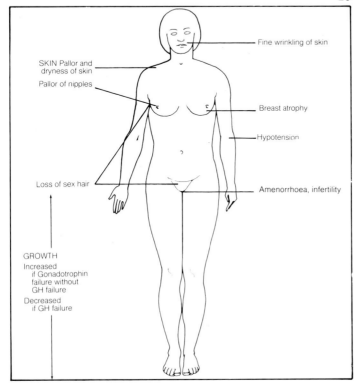

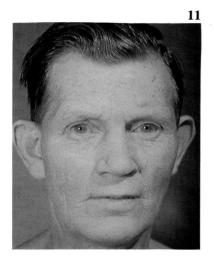

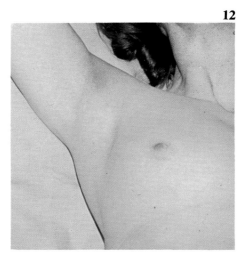

Gonadotrophin failure occurs early in pituitary failure and thus impotence in the male and amenorrhoea in the female are common early symptoms. The visual features include fine wrinkling of the skin round the mouth in both sexes (**11**), atrophy of genitalia and breasts and hair loss (**12**).

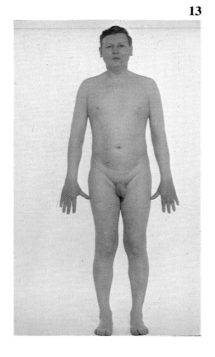

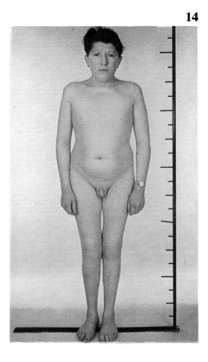

Gonadotrophin failure in childhood leads to failure to develop puberty (**13**) and if growth hormone secretion is normal, excessive linear growth. The presence of gonadotrophin failure can be confirmed by finding normal or low gonadotrophin levels in association with the clinical features described above.

Growth hormone deficiency leads to dwarfism (**14**) and delayed skeletal development in the child. Plumpness is common and fine wrinkling of the skin may be seen in the adult even if gonadotrophin deficiency is not present. Growth hormone deficiency can be confirmed by low growth hormone levels, which do not rise in response to hypoglycaemia, arginine, exercise or Bovril (meat extract).

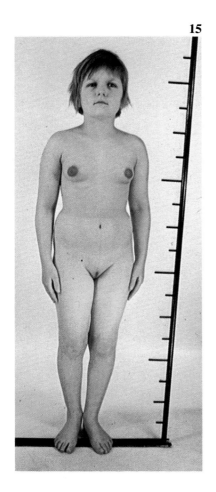

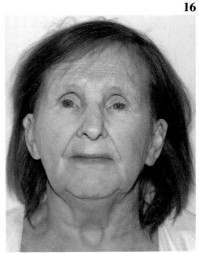

The clinical features of TSH deficiency in adults are those of hypothyroidism and include dryness of the skin, although the tissues do not generally become as coarse and thickened as in primary hypothyroidism (**16**). TSH deficiency may be difficult to recognise clinically. The diagnosis is confirmed by finding low thyroid hormone levels without an elevated TSH.

Thyrotrophin deficiency may contribute to growth retardation in children (**15** a child of 16 years).

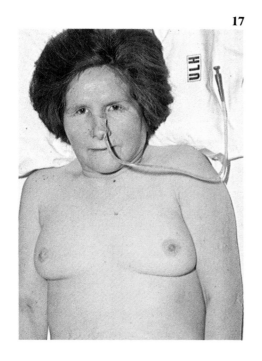

Adrenocorticotrophic hormone (ACTH) deficiency is generally slow in onset leading to weakness, nausea, hypoglycaemia, and collapse and coma if severe. ACTH deficiency may contribute to pallor of skin and nipples (**17**). The diagnosis is confirmed by low cortisol (hydrocortisone) levels which do not rise in response to hypoglycaemia.

Acromegaly and gigantism

Acromegaly is the clinical condition which results from an increased circulating growth hormone (GH) concentration in the adult. Gigantism is its counterpart in childhood. The disease is usually insidious in onset and slow to progress. **18** to **23** show a patient at 15, 27, 31, 32, 35 and 36 years of age.

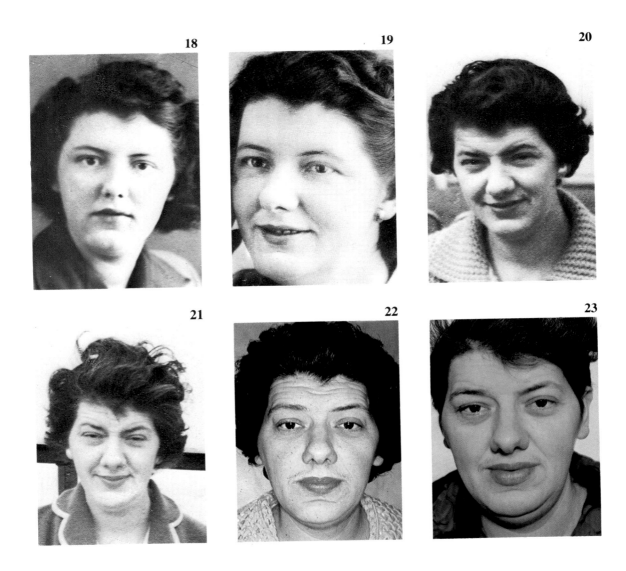

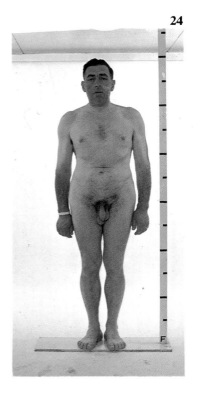

24

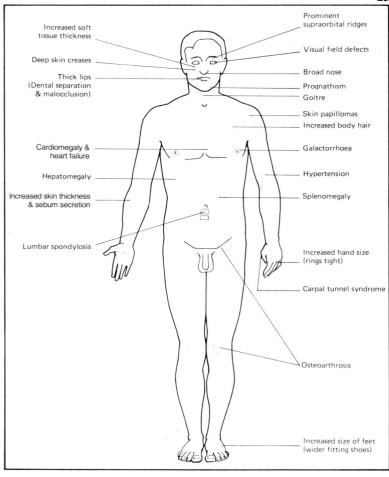

25

Increased soft tissue thickness

Deep skin creases

Thick lips (Dental separation & malocclusion)

Cardiomegaly & heart failure

Hepatomegaly

Increased skin thickness & sebum secretion

Lumbar spondylosis

Prominent supraorbital ridges

Visual field defects

Broad nose

Prognathism

Goitre

Skin papillomas

Increased body hair

Galactorrhoea

Hypertension

Splenomegaly

Increased hand size (rings tight)

Carpal tunnel syndrome

Osteoarthrosis

Increased size of feet (wider fitting shoes)

The presence of acromegaly is generally suspected from the typical clinical features (**24** and **25**), which include thickening of soft tissues and skin, broadening of the nose, increased prominence of supra-orbital ridges, prognathism (which may lead to dental malocclusion) and separation of the teeth (**26** and **27**).

26

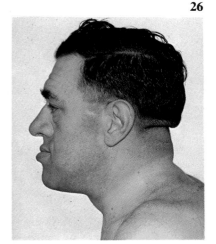

27

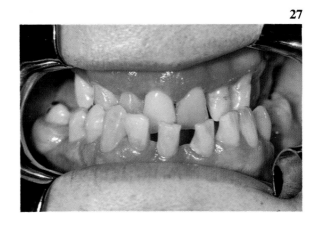

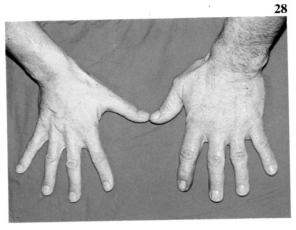

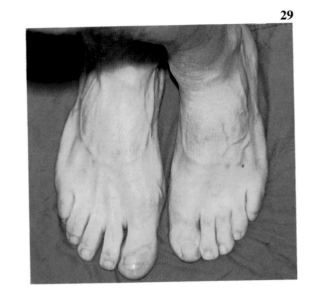

An increase in breadth of hands and feet is obvious. Rings may become tight and the patient requires progressively larger sizes of shoes. **28** and **29** show an acromegalic hand and foot compared with a normal hand and foot.

Finger size can be assessed by using jewellers' rings (**30**).

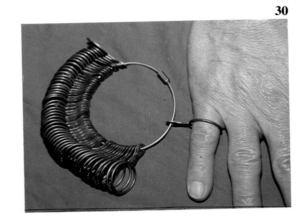

The hand provides a convenient site to assess skin thickness. The skinfold on the dorsum of the patient's hand can be compared with a skinfold on the dorsum of the examining hand (**31**).

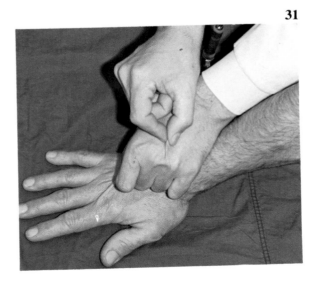

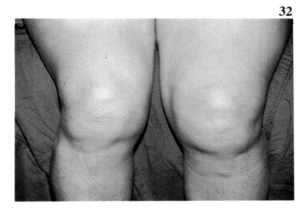

32

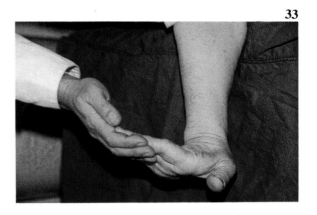

33

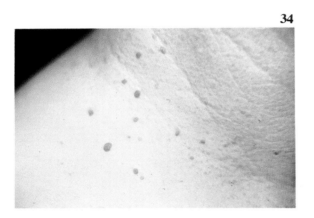

34

Other common clinical features include osteoarthrosis (**32** characterised by an increased joint space due to overgrowth of cartilage), increased laxity of ligaments (**33**), skin papillomata (**34**), acne (**35**) and heart failure (**36**), which may occur as a result of associated ischaemic heart disease, hypertension or cardiomyopathy.

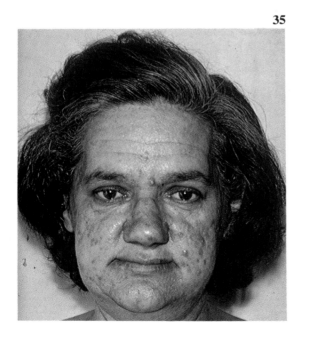

35

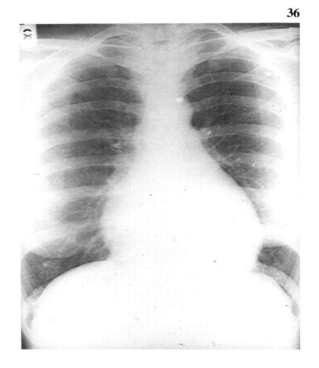

36

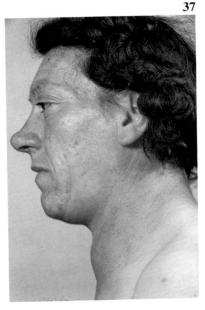

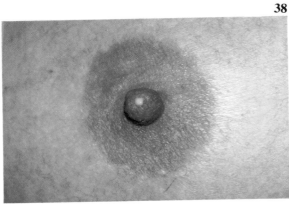

Galactorrhoea is not uncommon (**38**) and varying degrees of pituitary failure (due to expansion of the tumour) may be seen.

Enlargement of all the viscera is common. Hepatomegaly and splenomegaly may be found and goitre (**37**) is present in 20 per cent of patients.

Visual field defects may occur if the tumour extends outside the pituitary fossa. The most common defects are a bitemporal upper quadrantic defect or a hemianopia. **39** shows field defects in acromegaly.

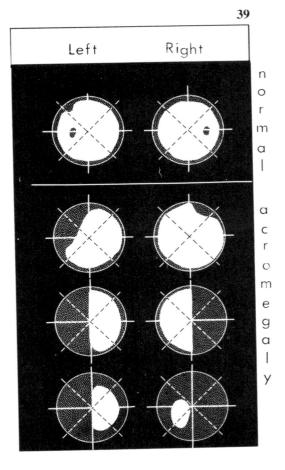

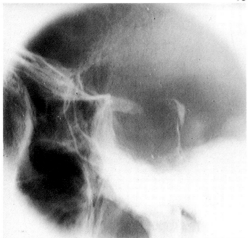

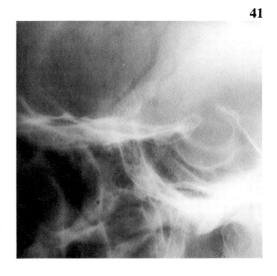

Expansion of the pituitary fossa is seen on a lateral skull X-ray in 90 per cent of patients (**40**). Asymmetry of the floor is often the earliest radiological sign (**41**). Abnormalities of the fossa may be found, with the aid of tomography, in 98 per cent of patients.

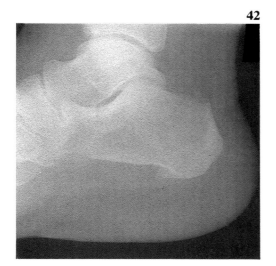

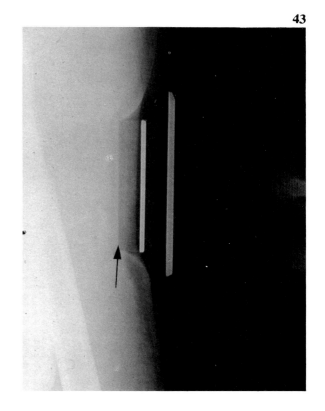

Increase in heel pad thickness (**42**) or skin thickness (**43**) may also be detected by appropriate radiological techniques.

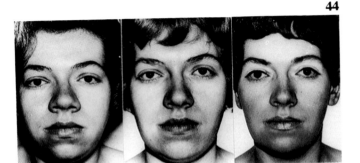

The diagnosis is confirmed by demonstrating an increase in GH level, which is not suppressed during a glucose tolerance test. The patient's appearance may improve significantly after treatment (**44**).

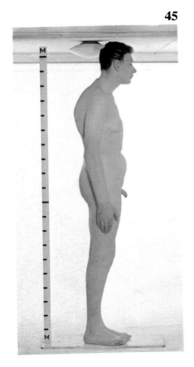

Gigantism results from increased circulating GH levels before epiphyseal fusion. A marked increase in linear growth is evident (**45**). The soft tissue changes are generally less evident, probably because of the age of the patients and the shorter period between onset and diagnosis.

Cushing's syndrome

The term 'Cushing's syndrome' describes those clinical disorders which result from an excess of circulating glucocorticoid. The term 'Cushing's disease' is currently used to describe those patients in whom the syndrome results from an increase in pituitary ACTH production. Bilateral adrenal hyperplasia is found in this group; this is the commonest cause (~90 per cent) of spontaneously occurring Cushing's syndrome. The clinical features are almost exclusively related to the increase in adrenal steroid production (**46**). This condition will, therefore, be considered with other disorders of the adrenal (pages 85–93).

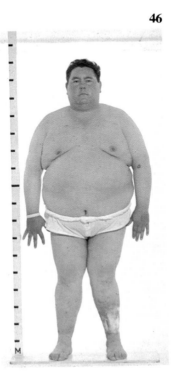

Galactorrhoea

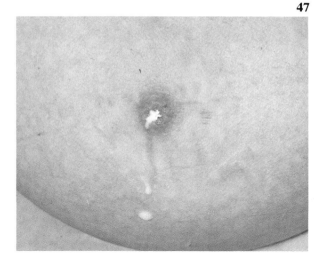

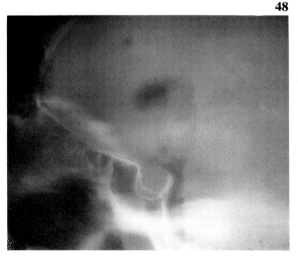

Galactorrhoea is lactation in the absence of an appropriate physiological stimulus (**47**). It may be unilateral or bilateral and may only be evident on expression. A serous or blood-stained discharge should always raise the possibility of an intrinsic breast lesion. Remember that some intraduct neoplasms cannot be detected by manual palpation.

No specific physical signs associated with galactorrhoea can be named, but there may be signs which suggest the presence of a pituitary tumour (**48** shows an enlarged pituitary fossa at air encephalography) or associated endocrine disease.

Causes of galactorrhoea

1 Hypothalamic or pituitary disease

Hypothalamic disturbance
Otherwise functionless adenomata
Cushing's disease
Acromegaly

2 Other endocrine disease

Primary hypothyroidism
Hyperthyroidism

3 Malignant disease

Oestrogen secreting tumours
Prolactin secreting tumours

4 Local disease or injury to the chest wall

5 Drugs

Oral contraceptives
Phenothiazines
Tricyclic antidepressants
Haloperidol
Methyl dopa
Reserpine

Diabetes insipidus

Diabetes insipidus occurs uncommonly in patients with pituitary disease. Simple destruction of the posterior lobe or pituitary stalk at worst only causes transient diabetes insipidus, because ADH is able to escape directly into the circulation from the axons of the hypothalamic neurones. A lesion has to be sufficiently large to produce considerable disturbance of the hypothalamus before diabetes insipidus occurs. Diabetes insipidus will be suspected in patients with a fluid intake and output greater than 3 litres in 24 hours.

49

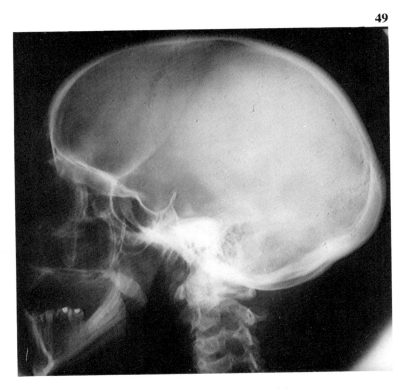

Diabetes insipidus is frequently associated with a craniopharyngioma and may be accompanied by other hypothalamic disturbance, sleep disorder, hyperphagia or hypophagia, disturbed thermostasis and inappropriate reduction in thirst, or altered emotional behaviour. **49** shows an X-ray of a craniopharyngioma with calcification.

The patient with polydipsia and polyuria may have primary polydipsia or primary polyuria.

Primary polyuria	Primary polydipsia
1 Impaired ability to secrete ADH Diabetes insipidus	Compulsive water drinking (Psychogenic polydipsia)
2 Target organ insensitivity to ADH Nephrogenic diabetes insipidus	Hypothalamic disease Hypokalaemia

3 Osmotic diuresis
   Diabetes mellitus
   Hypercalciuria
   Solute administration
	Hypercalcaemia

4 Renal tubular defects
   Chronic pyelonephritis
   Chronic renal failure
   Hypokalaemia
   Hypercalcaemia
   Sickle cell disease	

The investigation requires confirmation of a high fluid throughput, estimation of serum osmolality, and a fluid deprivation test.

Pituitary tumours

Pituitary tumours may be associated with acromegaly, gigantism, Cushing's disease, galactorrhoea or can be apparently non-secretory. The clinical importance of many pituitary tumours results from pressure upon normal pituitary tissue and adjacent structures, rather than their inherent secretory capacity. These may be chromophobe or chromophilic adenomas (50) and/or craniopharyngiomas (49). The latter may be detected radiologically by calcification in the tumour.

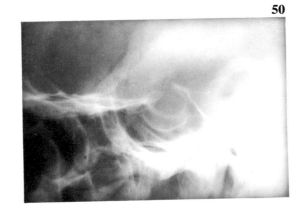

The more recent term 'functionless pituitary tumour' is open to question, because many are associated with excessive prolactin secretion (even though galactorrhoea may not be present). The extent of a pituitary tumour can be defined by an air encephalogram (51) or by computerised axial tomography. 52 shows suprasellar extension of a pituitary tumour. Compression of normal pituitary tissue may lead to impairment of endocrine function.

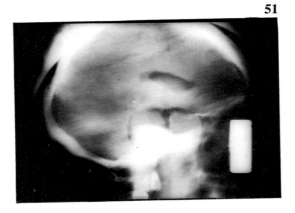

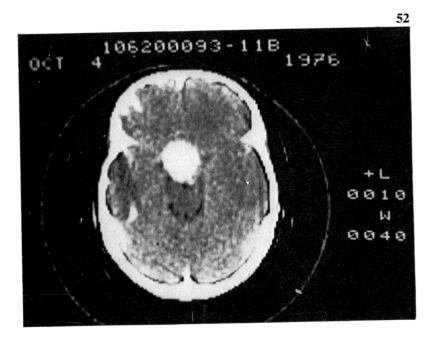

Visual field defects are present in a proportion of patients. A bitemporal upper quandrantic defect or hemianopia are most commonly seen (39).

53

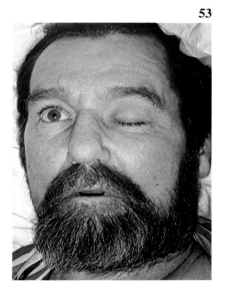

54

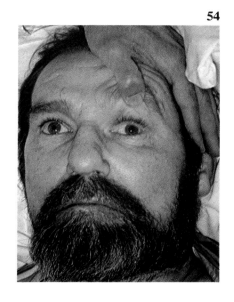

Asymmetrical expansion of the tumour occasionally leads to a unilateral field defect. Oculomotor palsies (53 and 54) are rare; papilloedema is very rare.

55

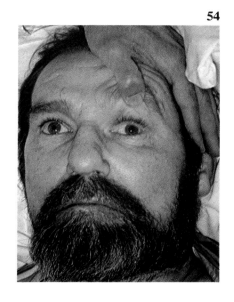

Optic atrophy (55) may result from long-standing suprasellar extension with compression of optic pathways.

2: Disorders of growth

Normal growth results from an interplay of many intrinsic and extrinsic factors on the innate genetically determined capacity for growth of the body cells. While growth and development proceed concomitantly in the normal child, these processes are to some extent potentially independent, and are under different hormonal and metabolic controls.

Although growth in height is most easily observed, alterations in skeletal proportions, maturation of the features, dental development and skeletal maturation must all be considered. The ultimate height attained depends not only on the rate of linear growth but on its duration, thus the actual height at a given age should always be assessed in the light of the bone maturity or bone age.

The clinical features which may be associated with short stature are shown in **1**.

1

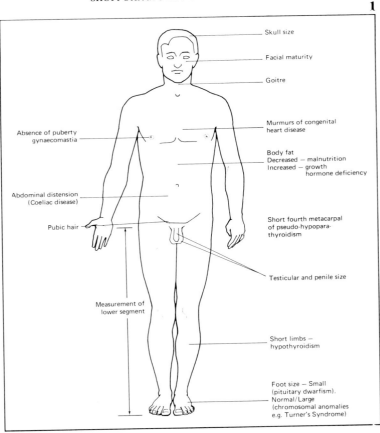

Skull size

Facial maturity

Goitre

Murmurs of congenital heart disease

Absence of puberty gynaecomastia

Body fat
Decreased — malnutrition
Increased — growth hormone deficiency

Abdominal distension (Coeliac disease)

Short fourth metacarpal of pseudo-hypopara-thyroidism

Pubic hair

Testicular and penile size

Measurement of lower segment

Short limbs — hypothyroidism

Foot size — Small (pituitary dwarfism). Normal/Large (chromosomal anomalies e.g. Turner's Syndrome)

Evaluation of growth

Height

Charts relating height to age indicate the rate of growth by comparison with a reference population. The most appropriate standards for height in the United Kingdom are the centile charts of Tanner and Whitehouse*. Midparental height charts allow correlation between a child's height and the mean height of both parents. When measurements of height are available over a whole year, they may be compared with normal by use of a growth velocity chart.

*A variety of growth charts are available from Castlemead Publications, Castlemead, Gascoyne Way, Hertford SG14 1LH.

Skeletal proportions

The lower segment, measured in the standing position, is the distance from the top of the symphysis pubis to the floor, the upper segment being obtained by subtraction of the lower segment from the total height. At birth the limbs, assessed by the lower segment, are relatively shorter but by 10 to 11 years of age, growth of the limbs causes the ratio of upper and lower segments to reach unity and the ratio is static into adult life.

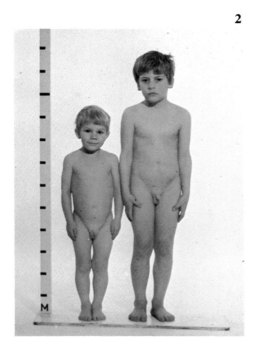

2

Hypothyroid dwarfs retain infantile proportions (unlike hypopituitary dwarfs and other types of dwarf, except those due to skeletal anomalies), and thus have a higher ratio of upper to lower segments. **2** shows a hypothyroid boy with age matched control. Measurement of the span is helpful because it largely reflects the length of the arms and is more than 5cm greater than the height in patients with eunuchoidal proportions e.g. Klinefelter's syndrome.

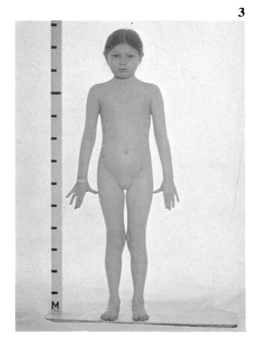

3

Weight

The relation of weight to age in the two sexes can be obtained from Tanner's charts. If growth is impaired by malnutrition, weight is likely to be reduced to a greater extent than height. **3** shows a malnourished short child with coeliac disease.

Maturation of features

Facial appearance is an important guide to skeletal maturity. Growth of the bridge of the nose is impaired during infancy in hypothyroidism and accounts for the characteristically immature face of the cretin (**4**).

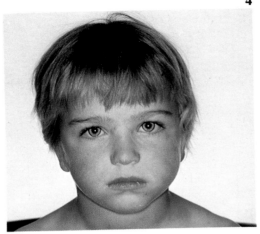

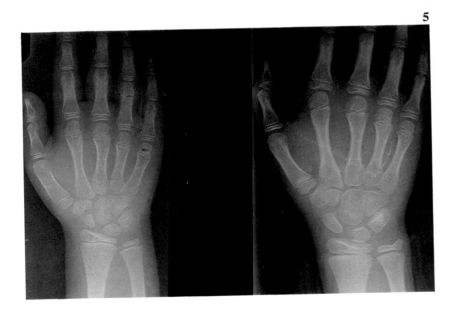

Bone maturation

Bone age is best determined by X-ray films of the hand and wrist which can be compared with plates depicting the degree of skeletal development of healthy children at different ages. For western communities the reader is referred to the *Radiographic Atlas of Skeletal Development of the Hand and Wrist* by W. W. Greulich and S. I. Pyle (1959). A skeletal age more than two standard deviations below the mean makes it highly probable that the child's bone maturation is abnormally retarded.

5 shows an X-ray of the left hand and wrist from a normal girl of 11 years of age (left) and an X-ray from a growth hormone deficient child of the same age and sex (right).

Dental development

This basic growth process may be assessed by inspection or by dental X-rays. Both primary and secondary dentition are affected by similar factors to those affecting bone maturation.

Short stature

Abnormal height cannot be defined absolutely, but a child is usually considered short if his height is below the third centile, which corresponds approximately to two standard deviations from the mean.

Most people of short stature are not suffering from endocrine or other disease. The cause can usually be determined by the clinical features and a few investigations. Particular attention should be paid to the family history of growth and development, the patient's birth weight and length, when available, the pattern of growth in height and epiphyseal development, facial features, secondary sexual characteristics, dental development, body weight, appetite and nutrition, infections and previous diseases, and intelligence. Clinical features which may be associated with short stature are shown in **1**.

Investigations may include urinalysis, blood count and erythrocyte sedimentation rate, chromosomal analysis (karyotype), X-rays of skull, chest, left hand and wrist (bone age), left knee (state of epiphyseal fusion), and other more specialised endocrine and metabolic tests as indicated.

Patients with abnormal proportions

Shortness of stature with abnormal proportions is uncommon but may cause gross stunting. Children with milder forms may be distinguished by comparing total height and sitting height, a measure of trunk length from Tanner's charts. The major types of short-limbed dwarfism are shown in Table **1** and figures **6** to **15**.

Table 1 Some types of short-limbed dwarfism*

Syndrome	Inheritance	Manifestations
Achondroplasia	Dominant	Large head and short limbs; distinct, milder types occur
Diastrophic dwarfism	Recessive	Limitation of joints; club foot; scoliosis develops after birth
Thanatophoric dwarfism	? Recessive	Very short limbs and small chest; all die in neonatal period
Achondrogenesis	Recessive	Grossly deficient calcification; all die in neonatal period
Conradi's syndrome	Recessive	Punctate calcification of developing cartilage
Spondyloepiphyseal dysplasia	Dominant and recessive	Several types; deformities become evident after birth
Metaphyseal dysostosis	Dominant	Tibial bowing; splayed metaphyses
Ellis–Van Creveld syndrome	Recessive	Chondroectodermal dysplasia with hypoplastic nails and teeth; congenital heart lesions
Cartilage-hair hypoplasia	Recessive	Fine, sparse, fragile hair; scalloped metaphyses
Hypophosphataemic rickets	X-linked dominant	Poor renal tubular reabsorption of phosphorus; need high dosage of Vitamin D
Hypophosphatasia	Recessive	Variable severity; low alkaline phosphatase levels
Osteogenesis imperfecta (fragilitas ossium)	Autosomal dominant (mutant)	Bowing of legs; pectus carinatum or excavatum; hyperextensible ligaments; kyphoscoliosis; hypoplastic teeth; thick skin; blue sclera; otosclerosis

*From Parkin, J. M., *Medicine*, 1975, **9**, 409

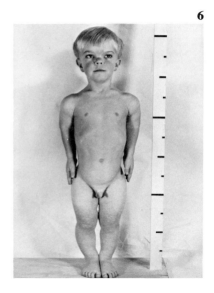

6

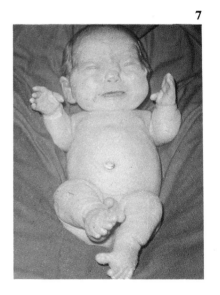

7

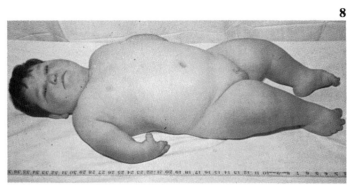

8

Bone disorders either acquired (some forms of *rickets*) or hereditary (*achondroplasia* **6**) are the main cause of this group of diseases. Other tissues may also be affected as shown in: *diastrophic dwarfism* (**7** and **8**) shown in the newborn and in an older child; *Conradi's syndrome* (**9** and **10**) showing an affected child and X-rays of the punctate calcification of developing cartilage.

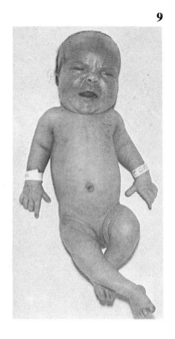

9

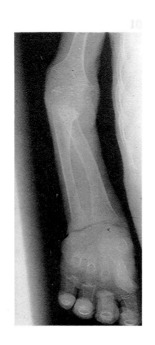

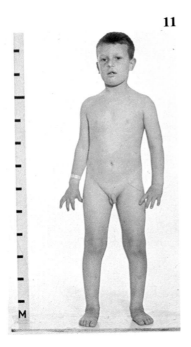

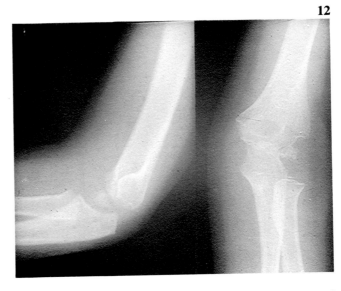

Epiphyseal dysplasia usually causes a mild form of short-limbed dwarfism. **11** and **12** show an affected child and an X-ray of the elbow in this condition.

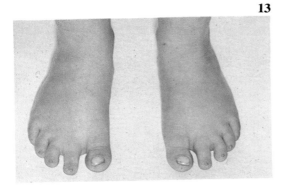

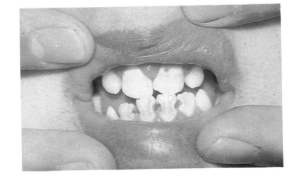

The *Ellis-Van Creveld syndrome* is a rare recessively inherited condition with chondroectodermal dysplasia with characteristic hypoplastic nails and teeth (**13** and **14**).

Osteogenesis imperfecta congenita may lead to shortness in severely affected cases sometimes with very short extremities (**15**). Physical examination and appropriate X-rays usually indicate that the basic problem involves the skeletal system.

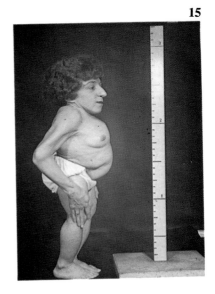

Patients with normal proportions

Those with normal proportions make up the major group of children with short stature.

Genetic causes Familial shortness may occur alone or be combined with delayed development, often also familial. This group is by far the commonest cause of short stature; diagnosis is usually easily established by a relevant family history. Charts correlating the child's height and the mid-parental height may be helpful (*vide supra*). Gross shortness is seen in the rare syndrome of *primordial dwarfism*.

16 and **17** show an affected child and an age and sex matched control.

16

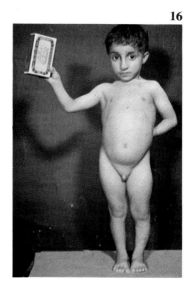

17

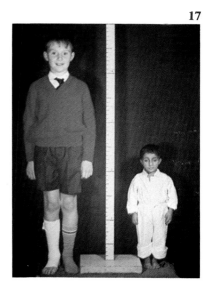

18

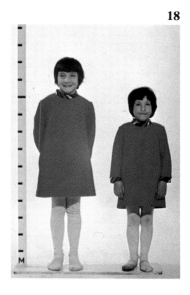

19

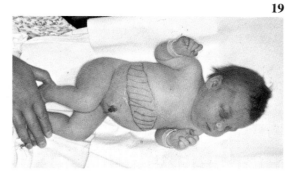

20

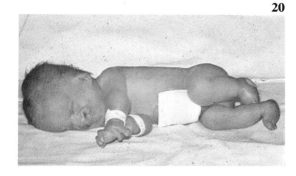

Low birth weight dwarfism constitutes a heterogenous group of children.

The unrecognised syndrome group comprises a wide variety of major and minor congenital anomalies including an odd facies, ptosis, an incurved fifth finger, or a high-arched palate.

An abnormal pregnancy producing an unhealthy placenta is a further cause of low birth weight dwarfism. Low birth weight dwarfism may lead to prolonged or even permanent shortness.

18 shows monozygotic twins of dissimilar birth weight at 7½ years of age.

Other cases include intrauterine infection, for example rubella or toxoplasmosis or chromosomal anomalies.

19 shows a child with intrauterine growth retardation caused by a congenital virus infection, rubella, which caused hepatosplenomegaly shown on skin markings, and thrombocytopenia. Autosomal chromosomal anomalies such as *Trisomy 9* (**20**) or one of the recognised or unrecognised syndromes, of which there are many, also cause intrauterine growth retardation.

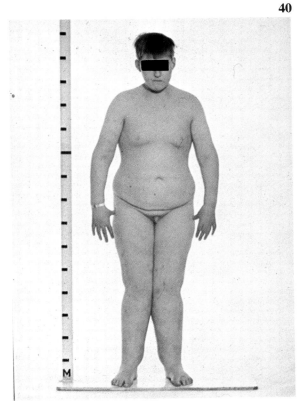

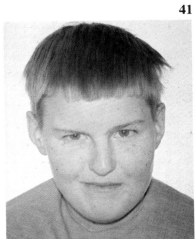

In the *Prader–Willi syndrome* (**40** to **42**) shortness, associated with gross obesity, mental retardation, small hands and feet, underdeveloped genitalia and later carbohydrate intolerance and diabetes mellitus are usually present.

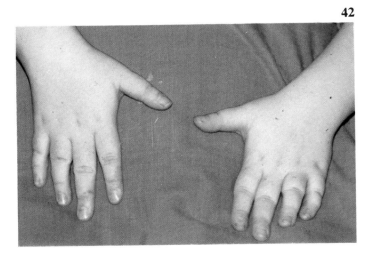

43

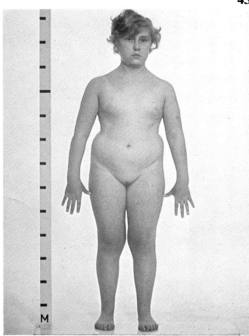

Sex chromosome anomalies These topics will be discussed in Chapter 5. *Turner's syndrome* (karyotype 45/XO) or its many chromosomal variants is always associated with short stature and delayed development. **43** shows a 16-year-old girl with short stature, primary amenorrhoea and lack of secondary sexual characteristics caused by XO/XY Turner's mosaicism. The characteristic somatic and radiological changes should be easily recognised.

Endocrine disorders Those disorders which cause shortness include congenital and acquired *deficiencies of growth hormone secretion and action* (see Chapter 1). The children are usually plump with immature facies and genitalia and delicate extremi-ties. **44** shows sibs, a 15-year-old boy and a 13-year-old girl with familial isolated growth hormone deficiency. **45** shows a 9-year-old pituitary dwarf compared with an age and sex-matched control.

44

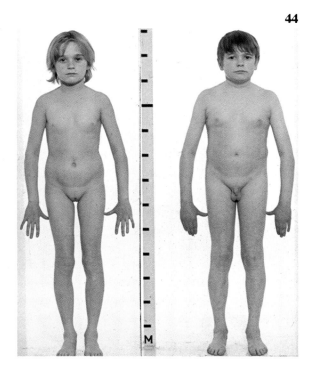

45

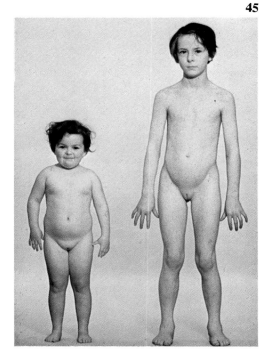

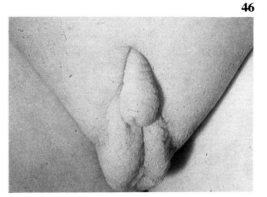

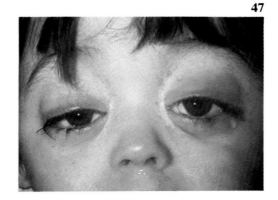

A micropenis (**46**) is present in one-third of boys with isolated growth hormone deficiency. Organic causes of GH deficiency include histiocytosis X, here shown affecting the orbit (**47**). Diabetes insipidus is frequently present as a result of hypothalamic deposits.

Hypothyroidism (see Chapter 3) should always be suspected in short children, the earlier its onset the more severe the deficit of skeletal length and maturation. Body proportions remain infantile and bone age is retarded more than height. **48**

shows a short hypothyroid child compared with an age and sex-matched control. **49** shows the wrist of a hypothyroid child aged three years with a bone age of six months.

48

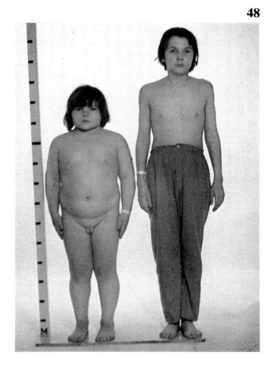

49

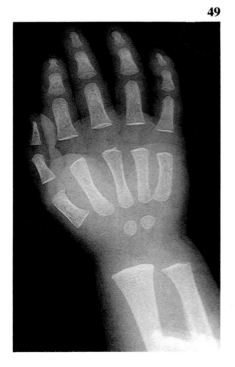

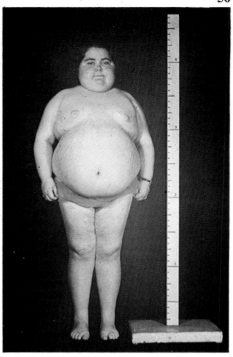

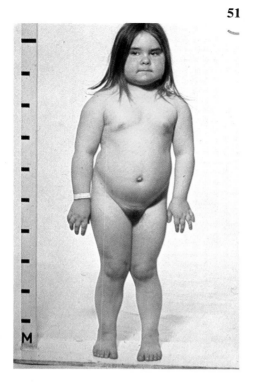

Cushing's syndrome (see Chapter 4)   In children this syndrome is always associated with growth retardation (**50**) and normal or even accelerated growth as seen in simple obesity rules out

Cushing's syndrome. **51** shows a short child with Cushing's syndrome caused by an adrenal adenoma associated with hemihypertrophy.

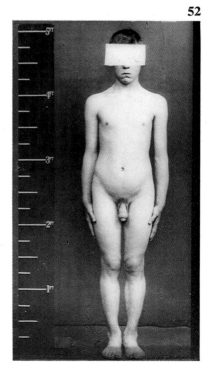

52

Congenital adrenal hyperplasia   Excessive androgen production (see Chapter 4) causes increased linear growth and skeletal maturation after birth. **52** shows a tall 10-year-old boy with precocious sexual development and hypertension caused by the 11ß-hydroxylase deficiency variety of congenital adrenal hyperplasia; however, the ultimate height is reduced.

Sexual prococity   Whether this is 'true' precocious puberty or caused by androgen or oestrogen secreting tumours, it is associated with excessive skeletal growth and maturation but a reduced ultimate height.

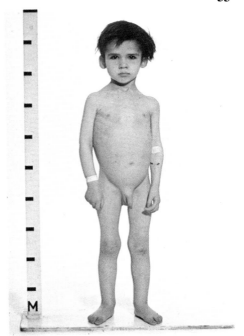

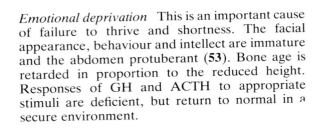

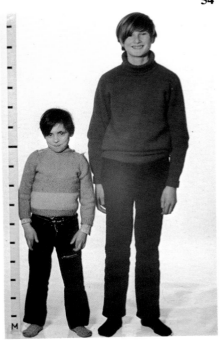

Emotional deprivation This is an important cause of failure to thrive and shortness. The facial appearance, behaviour and intellect are immature and the abdomen protuberant (**53**). Bone age is retarded in proportion to the reduced height. Responses of GH and ACTH to appropriate stimuli are deficient, but return to normal in a secure environment.

54 shows an emotionally deprived child with an age and sex-matched control.

Tall stature

Tall stature is a much less common medical problem than short stature, but it is appropriate to seek the cause in any child whose height is above the 97th centile.

Familial tall stature Most tall children and adults belong to this group, particularly if both parents are tall. They are well and their height falls within the normal range when allowance is made for mid-parental height, their growth running above but parallel to the 97th centile. Their ultimate height may be predicted from the tables of Bayer and Bayley* on the basis of their skeletal maturation.

---

*Bayer, L. M. and Bayley, N., *Growth Diagnosis*, University of Chicago Press, USA, 1959.

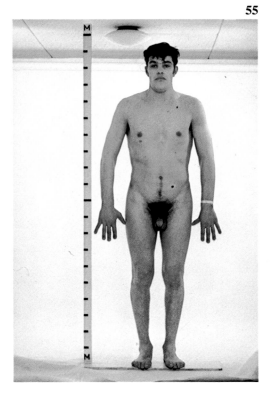

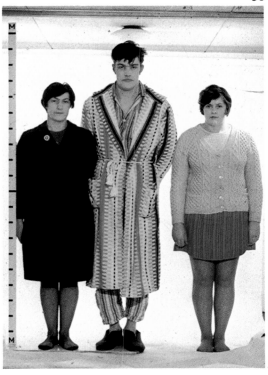

55 shows a tall man referred as possible acromegaly. When seen alongside his mother and sister he was clearly an example of familial tall stature (**56**).

Overnutrition Before puberty overnutrition tends to increase a child's height as well as weight but as bone age and puberty are also advanced, the adult height is not increased.

Advanced development This condition is the opposite of physiologically delayed puberty; it is often familial with rapid growth and advanced bone age throughout childhood, but a normal ultimate height is eventually achieved.

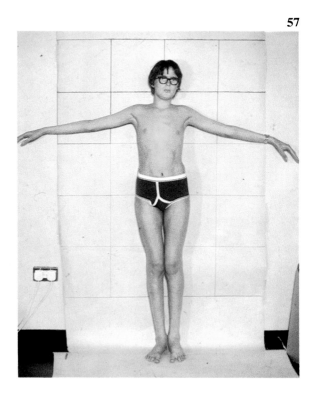

Syndromes A variety of syndromes causing tall stature may be recognised although most of these are rare. Children with generalised lipodystrophy may be tall. Patients with *Marfan's syndrome* (arachnodactyly) may be recognised by their numerous skeletal and somatic anomalies e.g. high arched palate, dislocated lenses, long fingers, toes and patellar ligaments, kyphoscoliosis, and pectus excavatum (**57** to **59**).

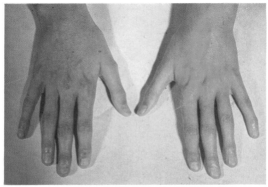

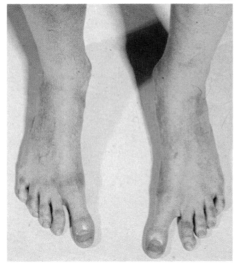

60

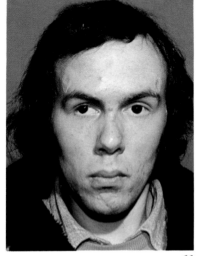

Sotos syndrome of cerebral gigantism is associated with clumsiness, mental retardation, macrocrania and prognathism, dolichocephaly, high arched palate, characteristic facies with frontal bossing, hypertelorism and antimongoloid obliquity of the palpebral fisures (**60** and **61**).

Chromosomal anomalies Patients with *Klinefelter's syndrome* (47/XXY) and with the 47/XYY syndrome (**62**) are usually tall. In the former at least this may be caused by androgen deficiency.

62

61

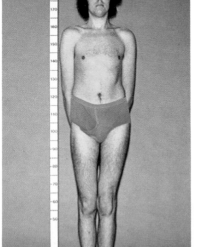

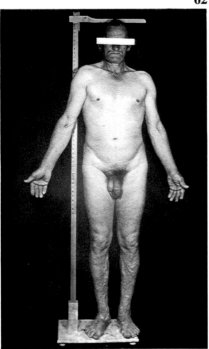

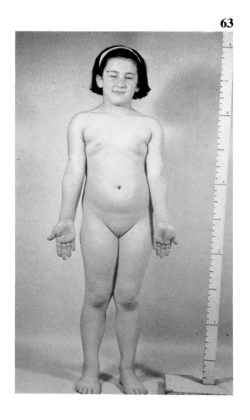

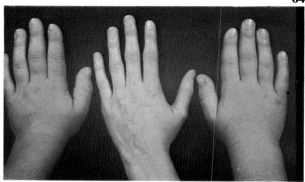

Hormonal Growth hormone excess from pituitary disease is very rare before puberty and some acromegalic features invariably accompany those of *gigantism*. **63** and **64** show a 4½-year-old girl with gigantism and features of acromegaly; her large broad hands are compared with those of a control.

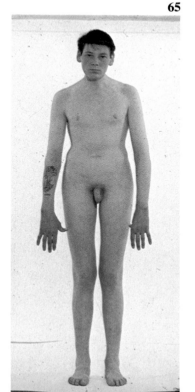

Sexual precocity Sexual precocity from any cause is initially accompanied by increased linear growth although the ultimate height is reduced.

Eunuchoidism – hypogonadism from any cause can produce an increase in growth caused by delayed fusion of epiphyses, so long as growth hormone secretion is maintained. This can be seen in solitary gonadotrophin deficiency with (Kallmann's syndrome) or without anosmia (**65**).

Hyperthyroidism In children hyperthyroidism produces an acceleration of growth rate with advanced bone age. Premature fusion of skull sutures can cause raised intracranial pressure.

3: Thyroid

Introduction

The thyroid gland secretes three hormones – thyroxine (T4), triiodothyronine (T3), and calcitonin. T4 and T3 are secreted by the follicular cells of the thyroid and calcitonin by the parafollicular or 'C' cells. The follicular cells are controlled by thyroid-stimulating hormone and possibly also by T4 and T3 themselves as part of a short-loop feedback. Calcitonin secretion is stimulated by elevation of the serum calcium level, but the role of calcitonin in normal physiology remains uncertain.

Clinical features of thyroid disease

The three common presentations of thyroid disease are:

1 Hyperthyroidism

2 Hypothyroidism

3 Goitre which may be non-toxic or associated with hypothyroidism or hyperthyroidism.

Hyperthyroidism

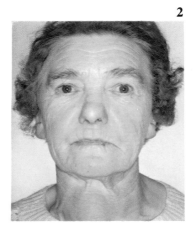

Hyperthyroidism is the clinical condition which results from increased circulating levels of thyroid hormone. The causes of hyperthyroidism include the following:

Graves' disease (**1**)
Toxic multinodular goitre (**2**)
Toxic adenoma (**3**)
Jod–Basedow phenomenon
Excess thyroid hormone ingestion
Molar hyperthyroidism
Pituitary hyperthyroidism
Viral thyroiditis (De Quervain's disease)
Ectopic hyperthyroidism

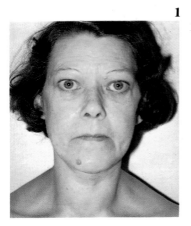

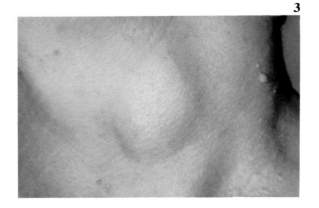

Graves' disease

This condition is the commonest form of hyperthyroidism seen in most western countries. It results from the action of thyroid-stimulating antibodies (TSAb) which interact with the TSH receptor. The major clinical features of Graves' disease are shown in 4 and include the following:

Hyperthyroidism
Goitre
Eye signs
Localised myxoedema
Thyroid acropachy
Other associated features

4

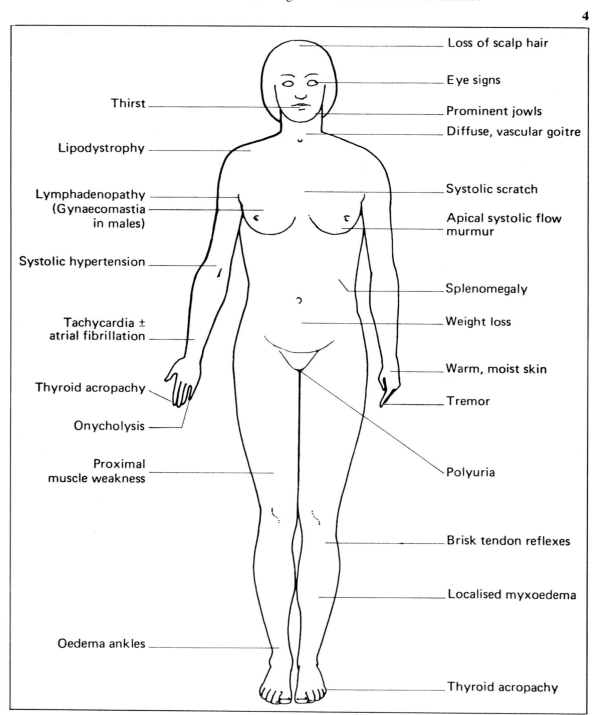

- Loss of scalp hair
- Eye signs
- Prominent jowls
- Diffuse, vascular goitre
- Systolic scratch
- Apical systolic flow murmur
- Splenomegaly
- Weight loss
- Warm, moist skin
- Tremor
- Polyuria
- Brisk tendon reflexes
- Localised myxoedema
- Thyroid acropachy

- Thirst
- Lipodystrophy
- Lymphadenopathy (Gynaecomastia in males)
- Systolic hypertension
- Tachycardia ± atrial fibrillation
- Thyroid acropachy
- Onycholysis
- Proximal muscle weakness
- Oedema ankles

Hyperthyroidism This condition may be associated with recession of the nails from the nail beds – onycholysis, the patient finding it difficult to keep her nails clean (5). The palms and fingers are warm and moist. A fine finger tremor is best appreciated by asking the patient to spread the fingers and rest them on the examiner's fingers (6).

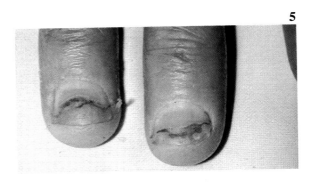

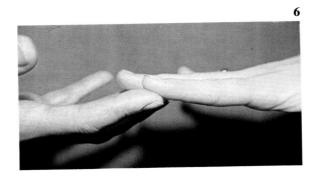

The pulse is usually rapid and forceful and, particularly in the elderly, atrial fibrillation may be present (7).
The systolic blood pressure may be elevated and the pulse pressure increased. Examination of the heart often reveals an apical systolic flow murmur and occasionally a squeaky exocardial scratch may be heard at the left sternal edge.

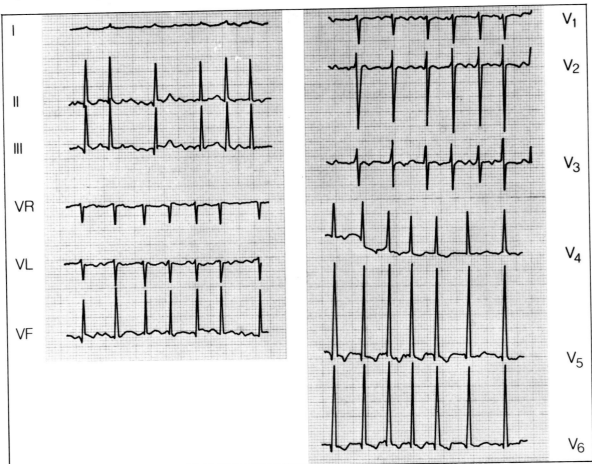

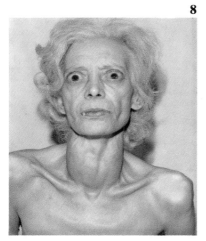

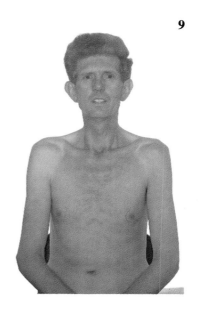

Weight loss may be apparent on inspection of the face (**8**) or trunk; muscle wasting may accompany a proximal myopathy (**9**). Splenomegaly and lymphadenopathy are seen in a few patients with long-standing disease. Ankle oedema is common even in the absence of heart failure.

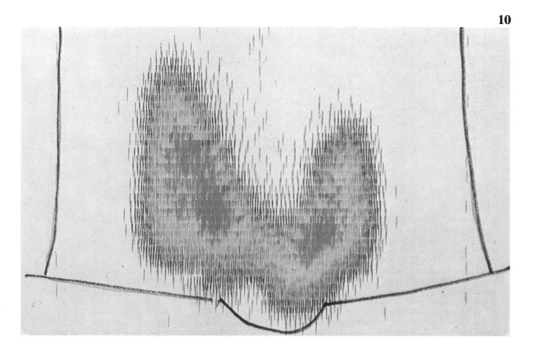

Goitre Enlargement of the thyroid gland is present in at least 90 per cent of hyperthyroid patients. In men the goitre may be less apparent, often being small, firm and close to the trachea. It is typical for the goitre to be diffusely enlarged and vascular. **10** shows a typical scan of the diffuse goitre of Graves' disease.

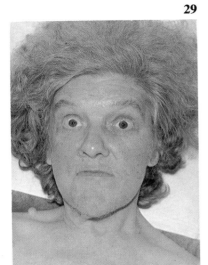

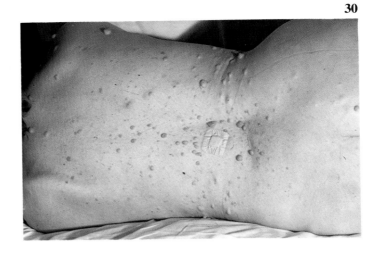

Usually some clinical evidence of the underlying pathology is present; for example, neurofibromatosis in a patient with a brain stem glioma (**29** and **30**).

Ptosis, not caused by myasthenia gravis, is a rare ocular feature of Graves' disease (**31**).

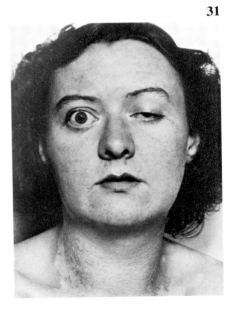

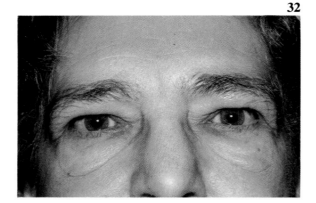

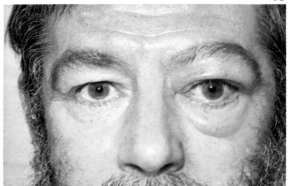

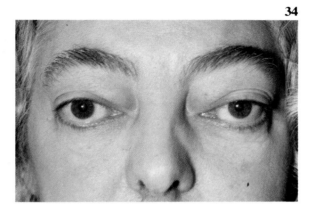

Periorbital swelling   This condition is common in Graves' disease when it may be unilateral or bilateral (**32**). It is often attributed to allergy affecting the lids, particularly when features of hyperthyroidism are absent. The periorbital swelling may have a slightly erythematous, oedematous appearance (**33**) or be caused by bulging of the orbital contents, usually fat, through the natural hiatuses of the anterior orbital septum (**34**) most obvious medially. The latter appearance can be seen in any space-occupying lesion affecting the orbit. The periorbital swelling of Graves' disease may be aggravated by that due to hypo-thyroidism in ophthalmic Graves' disease (**35**) or after destructive therapy to the thyroid.

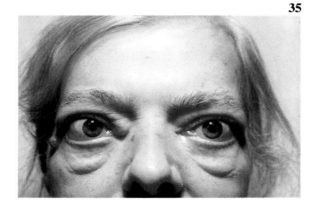

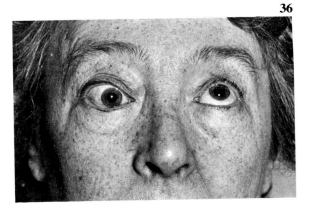

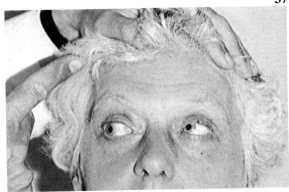

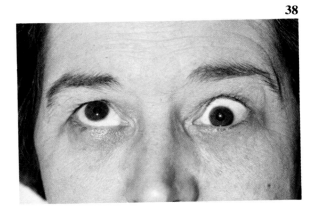

Ophthalmoplegia This condition which causes diplopia results from a characteristic pattern of lesions of the extraocular muscles. It may be suspected by the manner in which the patient tilts her head backwards in an effort to produce binocular vision. Tethering of muscles below the globe contributes to the defects in ocular movement, particularly upwards (36), which occur in a typical sequence. Upward and outward gaze is first affected (direction of movement mediated by the superior rectus) (37).

Upward and inward movement is next involved (direction of movement mediated by the inferior oblique) and later lateral gaze, medial gaze, and finally inferior gaze are affected.

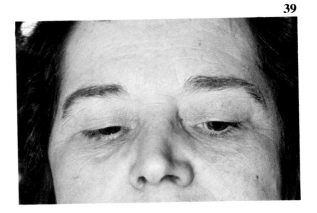

The latter three lesions occur in diminishing frequency and never without some defect in upward gaze which causes the patient more than the normal discomfort. Ophthalmoplegia affecting upward gaze may be accompanied by the paralytic variety of lid retraction.

Retraction of the upper lid is enhanced when the patient looks up (38) and is abolished when the patient looks down (39), in contrast with the commoner spastic variety of lid retraction which differs little with different directions of gaze.

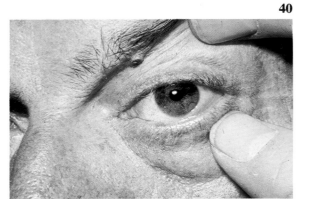

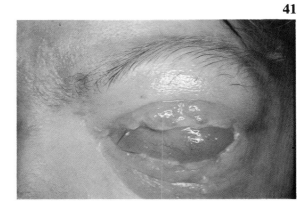

Chemosis, superficial punctate keratitis These are usually features of more severe ophthalmopathy. Chemosis can be mild (**40**) or so severe that

the oedematous conjunctiva prolapses between the lids (**41**).

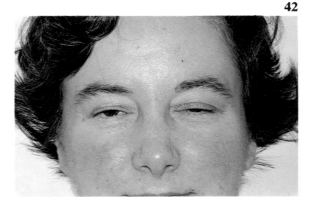

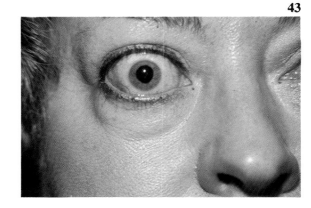

Superficial punctate keratitis or more severe corneal ulceration cause pain or discomfort in the eyes with lacrimation and sometimes blepharo-

spasm (**42**). Injection over the insertions of the extraocular muscles is common in severe ophthalmopathy (**43**).

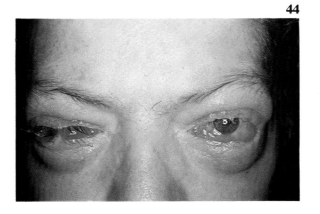

'Congestive ophthalmopathy' This term should be used in place of 'malignant exophthalmos' because the word 'malignant' may alarm the patient; exophthalmos may not be present in some patients with this sight-threatening complication. The eyes are 'active' and inflamed, chemosis is invariably present and the medial caruncles are swollen and may prolapse between the lids (**44**). Ophthalmoplegia is invariably present as is periorbital swelling, although the more typical ocular features of exophthalmos and lid retraction may be absent or trivial. There are a variety of causes of visual failure in congestive ophthalmopathy.

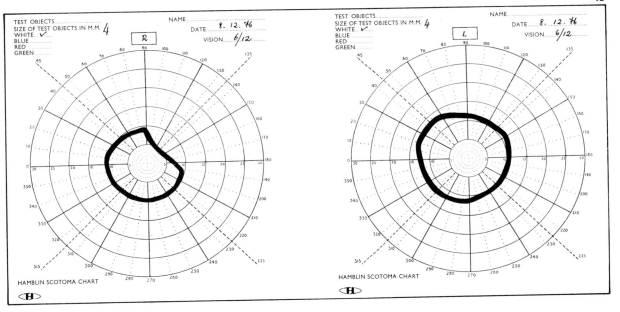

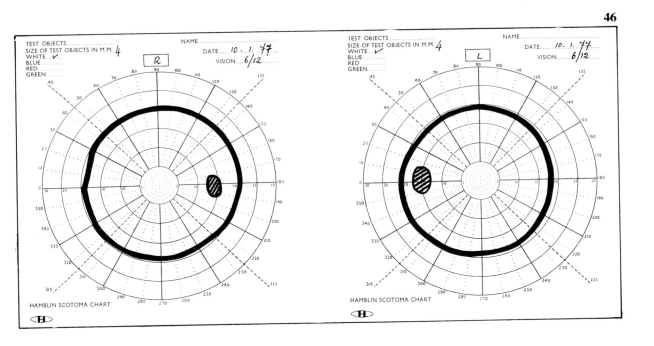

Corneal ulceration from exposure is a major hazard. Glaucoma is occasionally associated. Optic-nerve compression may cause a defect in red-green colour vision in the absence of papilloedema; concentric field defects often remain unrecognised. **45** and **46** show concentric field defects occurring in congestive ophthalmopathy and their subsequent improvement as a result of dexamethasone therapy.

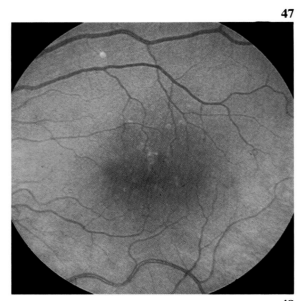

Macular oedema (47) causes defects of visual acuity in some patients. Refractive errors resulting from compression of the globe by the swollen orbital contents can be corrected by appropriate lenses, and should not be mistaken for optic-nerve compression.

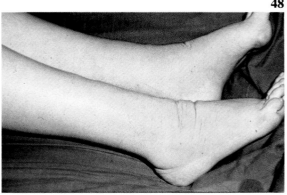

Localised myxoedema usually affects the shins (48) or top of the feet but may be seen on the face, hands or back, unusual sites which may sometimes be determined by local pressure or trauma. Several varieties of localised myxoedema may be recognised.

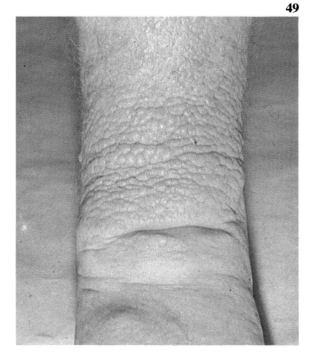

The typical form of localised myxoedema consists of a sheet of thickened cutaneous or subcutaneous tissue of pink or violaceous hue, with coarse hairs and little pitting (48, 49).

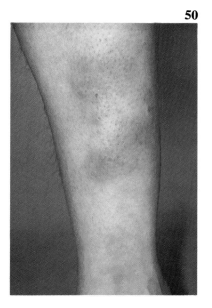

50

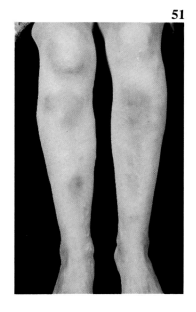

51

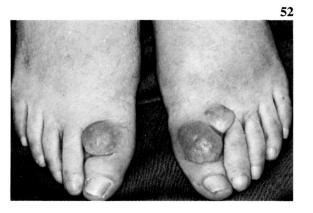

52

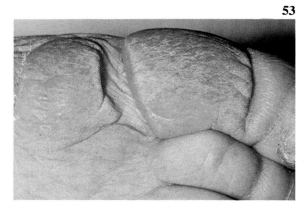

53

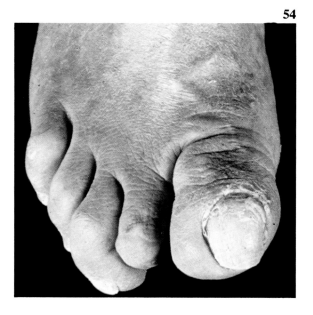

54

The nodular form of localised myxoedema (**50**) has a similar appearance to erythema nodosum (**51**), but is non-tender or only slightly so. Although this variety is quite common, it is often overlooked. Spontaneous remission is the rule. Occasional horny nodules develop on the dorsum of the toes especially the big toe (**52** and **53**). This must be differentiated from pachyderma periostitis (**54**).

The oedematous form of localised myxoedema simulates venous oedema of the legs or ankles, pitting is present, the skin is little thickened yet biopsy reveals typical histological and histo-chemical features of localised myxoedema.

55

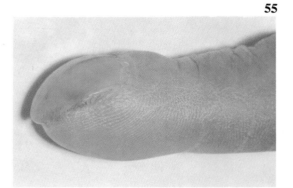

56

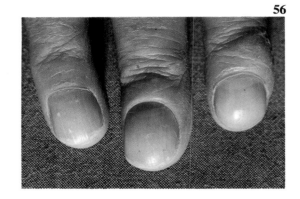

57

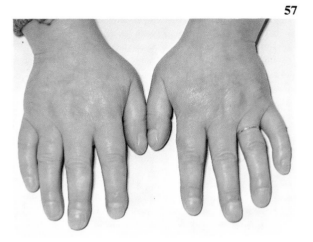

58

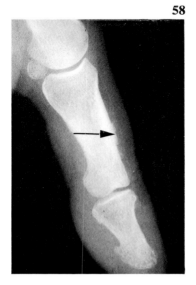

59

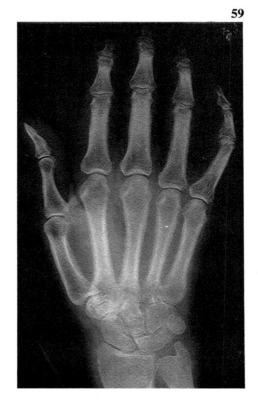

Thyroid acropachy resembles clubbing of the fingers and toes (**55**), but the oedema of the nail folds seen in the latter is inconspicuous and the thumb and index fingers are most severely involved (**56** and **57**). X-ray of the hands and wrists may show patchy sub-periosteal new bone formation resembling bubbles (**58**); this differs from the linear new bone formation seen in hypertrophic osteoarthropathy (**59**).

Other associated features of Graves' disease

Among these features are prominent jowls, gynaecomastia, splenomegaly, vitiligo, and myasthenia gravis.

60 **61**

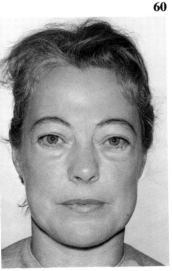 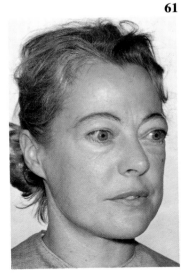

Prominent jowls may be seen in patients with Graves' disease usually accompanied by exophthalmos and localised myxoedema. This is caused by an abnormal distribution of fat over the mandible, just below the angle of the jaw (**60** and **61**).

Gynaecomastia, usually without galactorrhoea, is seen in some men with Graves' disease.

Splenomegaly is an uncommon association and alternative causes should be considered.

62

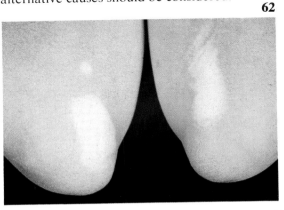

63

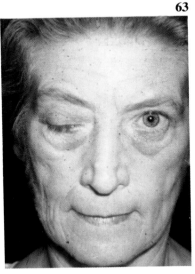

Vitiligo is a cutaneous marker of the organ specific autoimmune diseases (**62**).

63 shows ptosis in a patient with myasthenia and Graves' disease.

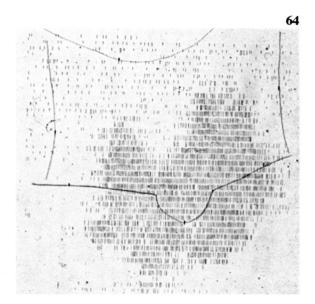

64

Toxic multinodular goitre

Toxic multinodular goitre is commoner in areas of iodine deficiency, particularly after the introduction of iodised salt (Jod–Basedow phenomenon). The condition may represent autonomous hyperfunction of a varying number of nodules when the appearance of the thyroid scan is characteristic (**64**) and eye signs are absent. Alternatively, typical Graves' disease may occur in a patient with a pre-existing nodular goitre.

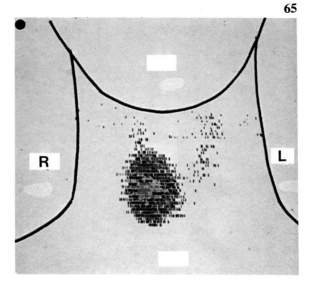

65

Toxic adenoma

Autonomous function of one or more thyroid adenomas may cause hyperthyroidism, or the excess of thyroid hormones may only be sufficient to suppress pituitary TSH secretion and reduce the function of the rest of the thyroid without causing clinical evidence of hyperthyroidism (subclinical toxic adenoma).

The appearance of the thyroid scan is characteristic (**65**); uptake over the nodule is not suppressed by triiodothyronine administration, but uptake of the rest of the gland can be enhanced by thyroid-stimulating hormone. Such hot nodules are very rarely malignant.

Hypothyroidism

Hypothyroidism is the clinical condition which results from decreased circulating levels of thyroid hormones. It may be classified as primary when resulting from diseases of the thyroid, secondary when hypothalamic or pituitary disease is responsible, and peripheral when, very rarely, it results from a decreased tissue responsiveness to thyroid hormones.

Primary hypothyroidism may be caused by the following:

Athyreosis or hypoplasia
Ectopic thyroid
Endemic cretinism
Endemic iodine deficiency
Dyshormonogenesis
Drug administration
Autoimmune thyroid disease
Post-destructive therapy for hyperthyroidism or carcinoma

The pituitary thyroid relationships in primary hypothyroidism are shown (**66**). Primary hypothyroidism is characterised by lowered circulating levels of thyroid hormones and a raised level of thyroid-stimulating hormone.

66

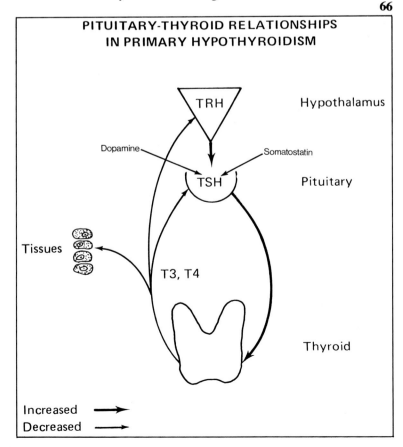

PITUITARY-THYROID RELATIONSHIPS IN PRIMARY HYPOTHYROIDISM

TRH — Hypothalamus
Dopamine
Somatostatin
TSH — Pituitary
Tissues
T3, T4
Thyroid
Increased →
Decreased →

Neonatal hypothyroidism

In non-endemic goitre areas the condition results from absence of the thyroid (athyreosis), ectopic thyroid, dyshormonogenesis, drug administration, or more rarely from isolated pituitary TSH de-ficiency. The condition is found in about 1/4000 births in areas where iodine deficiency is not endemic. The clinical features of cretinism are only rarely recognised before the age of six weeks.

67

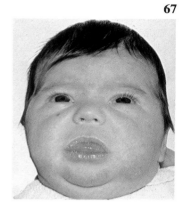

68

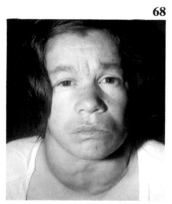

Prolonged neonatal jaundice may provide a clue to the diagnosis, although most children with neo-natal jaundice do not suffer from hypothyroidism. The characteristic facial appearance of the cretin (**67**) with protruding tongue and coarse features may not be obvious until several months after birth, and there are other causes of mental retarda-tion and umbilical hernia. Neurological complica-tions are common in endemic cretins some of whom have obvious goitres (**68**).

69

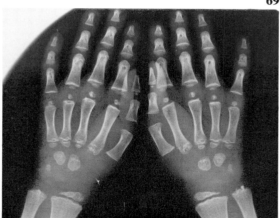

70

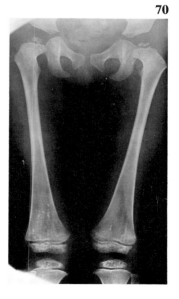

The bony changes of cretinism include delayed bone age, widening of the epiphyseal line, deformed epiphyses, abnormal bone texture and irregularity of the metaphyses. Most of these features are shown in the hand X-rays of a 12-year-old cretin (**69**). There may be a thoraco-lumbar kyphosis with deformed vertebrae and a brachycephalic skull with delayed closure of the fontanelles.

Epiphyseal dysgenesis, an appearance of frag-mentation of the epiphysis, can be seen here affecting the femoral head (**70**).

Endemic iodine deficiency hypothyroidism

Hypothyroidism from iodine deficiency in an endemic goitre area may present at any age; the clinical features differ in no way from those of hypothyroidism occurring in a non-endemic area, apart from the presence of a goitre.

71

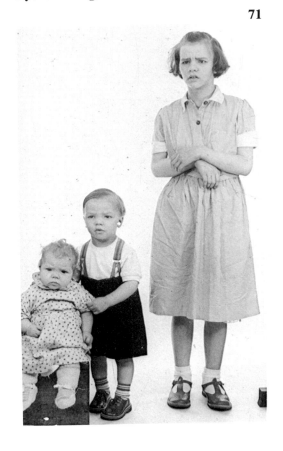

72

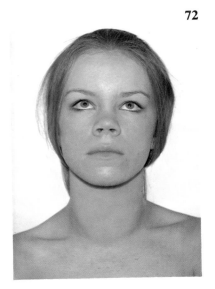

A variety of thyroidal enzyme defects result in goitre and hypothyroidism of varying degrees of severity. The condition is usually familial (**71**), presents in childhood and may be associated with nerve deafness (Pendred's syndrome, **72**) and mental retardation.

73

Drug administration

A variety of drugs (goitrogens) cause impairment of thyroid hormone synthesis which leads to thyroid enlargement and, if compensation is inadequate, to hypothyroidism. Occasionally hypothyroidism can occur without goitre. The drugs responsible vary in different parts of the world, depending on habits of prescribing and self-administration.

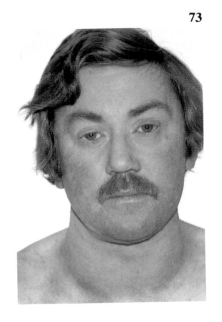

In the UK iodides taken as constituents of cough medicines and proprietary asthma preparations are common causes of drug-induced goitre (**73**). The association of these thyroid disorders with chest disease should always alert the clinician to the possibility of iodide goitre.

74

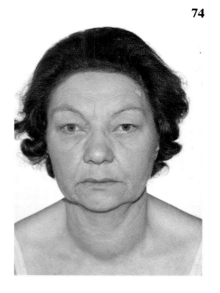

This condition is the commonest cause of spontaneous hypothyroidism in most western countries. Hypothyroidism caused by autoimmune thyroid disease may be associated with a goitre, but frequently the thyroid is small although firm, or impalpable. The term 'Hashimoto's disease' can be used to describe patients with a diffusely enlarged, firm, finely nodular goitre, who may be euthyroid or have any degree of thyroid failure (**74**).

Autoimmune thyroid disease may be suspected if there is a personal or family history of diabetes mellitus, pernicious anaemia, or autoimmune thyroid disease.

Other conditions associated with autoimmune thyroid disease include the following:

Vitiligo – recognised by patchy, symmetrical depigmentation of the skin surrounded by areas of increased pigmentation (**75**).

Alopecia areata – patchy loss of scalp hair (**76** and **77**).

75

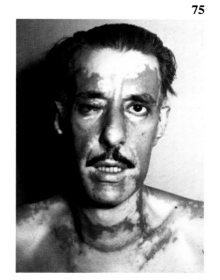

77

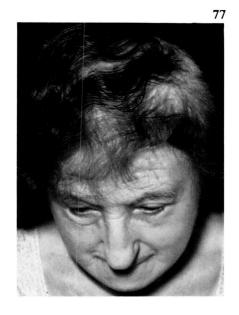

76

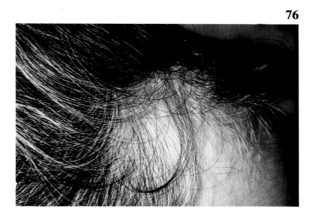

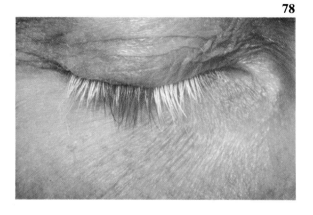

78

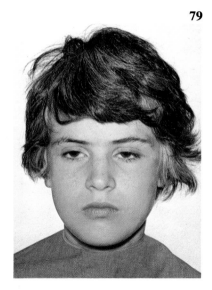

79

Leucotrichia – white patches of hair affecting the scalp, eyelashes (**78**) or body hair.

Premature greying of the hair – seen characteristically in pernicious anaemia but also in the auto-immune thyroid diseases. **79** shows an 11-year-old girl with greying hair.

Halo naevi – where a pigmented naevus gradually loses its pigmentation (**80**).

Hypothyroidism

This condition may be of any degree of severity from overt, myxoedema (**81**), through mild hypothyroidism (**82**) where the clinical features are slight and easily mistaken for the natural process of ageing, to subclinical hypothyroidism where there are no clinical manifestations but an elevated serum TSH level.

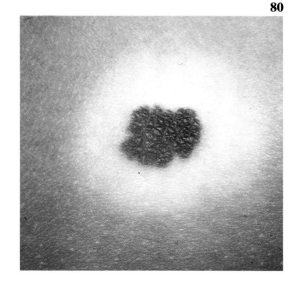

80

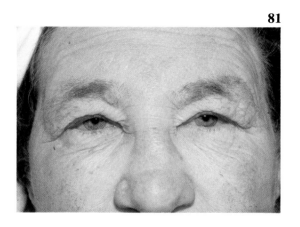

81

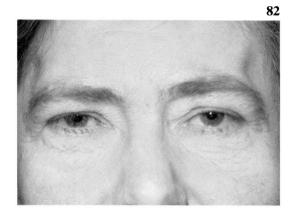

82

The characteristic clinical features of hypothyroidism are shown in **83** and include the following. Coarsening and loss of scalp and body hair (**84**), puffiness of the face with periorbital swelling which may be mild or very obvious (**85**).

83

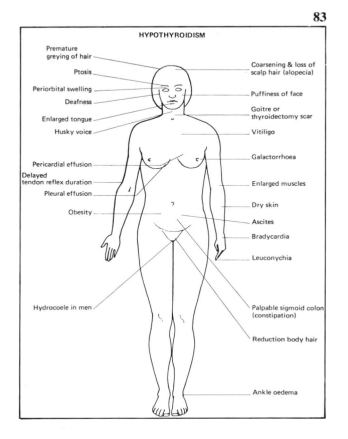

HYPOTHYROIDISM

Premature greying of hair

Ptosis

Periorbital swelling

Deafness

Enlarged tongue

Husky voice

Pericardial effusion

Delayed tendon reflex duration

Pleural effusion

Obesity

Hydrocoele in men

Coarsening & loss of scalp hair (alopecia)

Puffiness of face

Goitre or thyroidectomy scar

Vitiligo

Galactorrhoea

Enlarged muscles

Dry skin

Ascites

Bradycardia

Leuconychia

Palpable sigmoid colon (constipation)

Reduction body hair

Ankle oedema

84

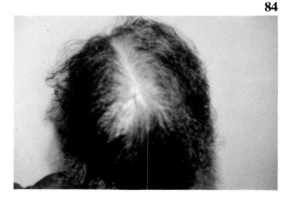

85

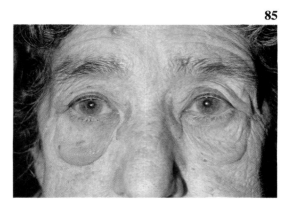

86

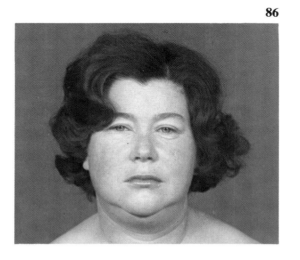

87

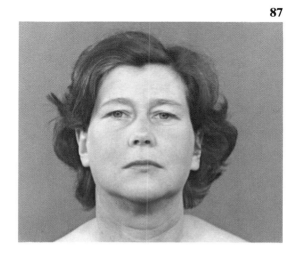

The improvement in appearance resulting from therapy is well shown in **86** and **87**.

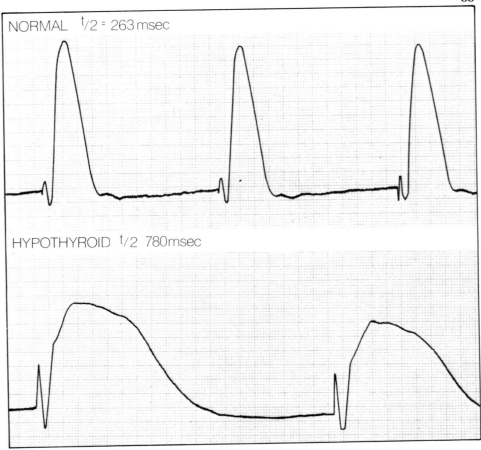

NORMAL $t/2$ = 263 msec

HYPOTHYROID $t/2$ 780 msec

Delay in the relaxation phase of the tendon reflexes can be measured as the Achilles tendon reflex duration time (**88** shows normal and hypothyroid patterns) and observed clinically by gentle percussion of the biceps tendon.

The ECG changes of hypothyroidism include bradycardia, reduced voltage of P, R and T waves and inversion of the T waves, changes which soon resolve with thyroid hormone treatment (**89**).

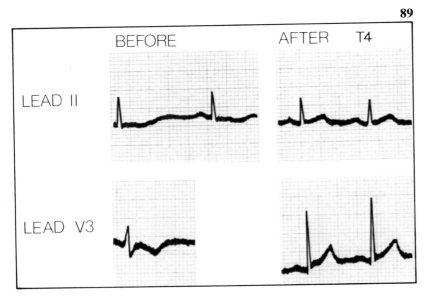

BEFORE   AFTER   T4

LEAD II

LEAD V3

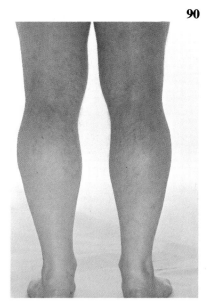

90

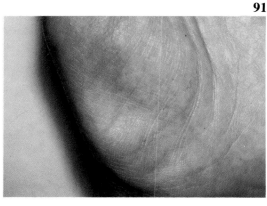

91

Muscle enlargement (**90**) may be associated with a visible lump on percussion over the body of the muscle. Wasting of the thenar eminence may result from long-standing median nerve compression in hypothyroidism (**91**).

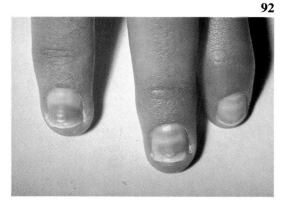

92

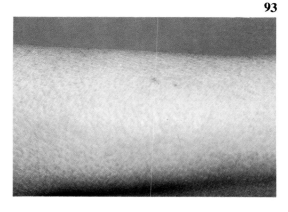

93

Leuconychia (**92**), white nails are also associated with cirrhosis. Dryness of the skin may be best observed by inspecting the forearm tangentially

(**93**) and should be differentiated from congenital xeroderma.

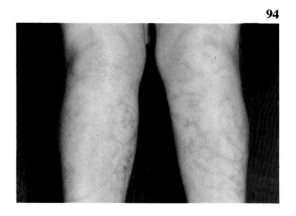

94

Erythema ab igne (**94**) may result from the patient sitting too close to a fire.

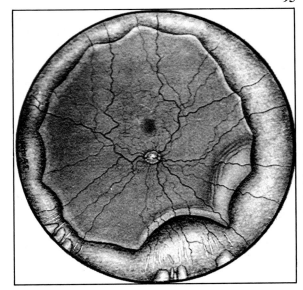

Effusions into body cavities may be observed.

a) Uveal effusions seen on fundoscopy (**95**) may impair vision.
b) Middle and inner ear effusions may contribute to the deafness, unsteadiness and sometimes true vertigo seen in hypothyroidism.
c) Pericardial effusions (**96** and **97**, chest X-rays showing a pericardial effusion and its resolution after thyroxine therapy) and pleural effusions.

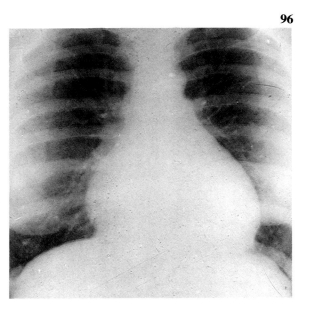

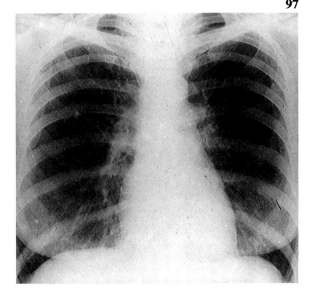

d) Ascites (**98**).
e) Joint effusions are uncommon.
f) Hydroceles may be seen which remit after therapy of the hypothyroidism.

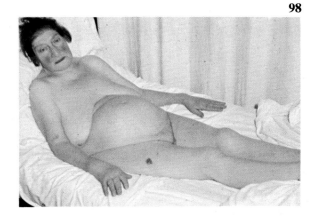

99

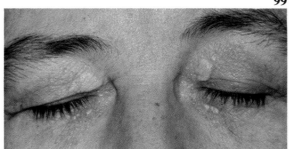

Xanthelasma may occasionally complicate the long-standing hypercholesterolaemia associated with hypothyroidism (**99**).

100

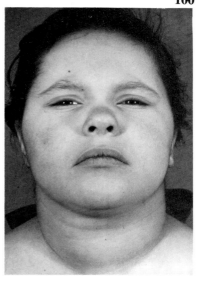

101

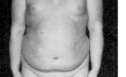

Features of juvenile hypothyroidism

There are a number of features either peculiar to or which occur more commonly in juvenile hypothyroidism.

Shortness of stature Hypothyroidism should always be excluded in a short child or adolescent. **100** and **101** show a short hypothyroid girl before thyroxine and **102** and **103** after therapy.

102

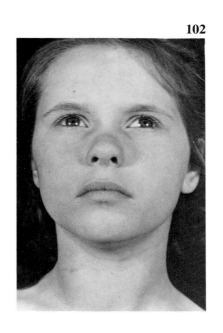

103

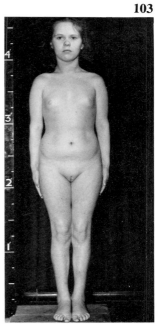

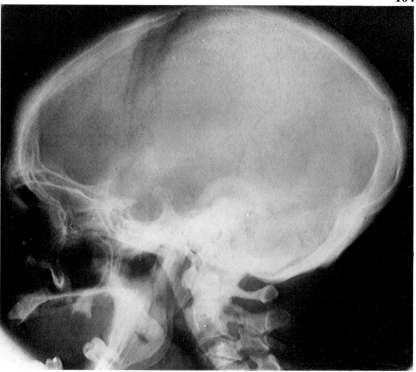

Enlargement of the pituitary fossa from feedback hyperplasia or tumour formation of the thyrotroph cells is seen in some cretins, but also in adults with long-standing untreated hypothyroidism (**104**). *Precocious puberty* is a rare association of juvenile hypothyroidism. *Galactorrhoea* can be seen in hypothyroid children or adults. *Pigmentation of the skin* is another feature of juvenile hypothyroidism.

Goitrous hypothyroidism

This condition is seen in Hashimoto's disease, dyshormonogenetic goitre, after drug administration, and in iodine deficient areas.

Risk factors for hypothyroidism

A large number of patients exhibit non-specific symptoms and signs which would be compatible with hypothyroidism, but certain risk factors make it worthwhile to consider a diagnosis of hypothyroidism in an individual patient.

Family history A family history of goitre or hypothyroidism in a child raises the possibility of dyshormonogenesis. In an adult a positive personal or family history of organ-specific auto-immune disease e.g. pernicious anaemia or diabetes mellitus is helpful.

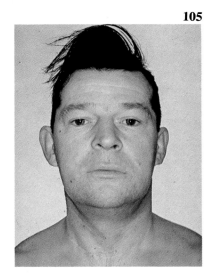

Goitre or a thyroidectomy scar This indicates the presence of thyroid disease and hypothyroidism is always a possibility (**105**).

Vitiligo, premature greying of the hair, leucotrichia and alopecia areata, as mentioned previously, are associated with the organ-specific autoimmune diseases and hence with hypothyroidism or hyperthyroidism.

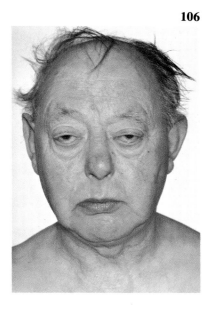

Eye signs of Graves' disease Patients with Graves' disease may develop hypothyroidism either spontaneously or as a result of destructive therapy. **106** shows a patient with overt hypothyroidism after a thyroidectomy 30 years before with residual eye signs of Graves' disease.

Goitre

Enlargement of the thyroid is referred to as a goitre. The problem facing the clinician when a patient complains of a swelling in the neck is to decide whether or not the thyroid is enlarged. A normal thyroid gland in a male is rarely palpable, but in a woman with a thin neck one can often feel the gland. Observer variation in assessment of thyroid size is considerable, particularly in deciding whether the thyroid is normal yet just palpable or there is a small goitre. Pads of fat over the front of the neck may simulate thyroid enlargement.

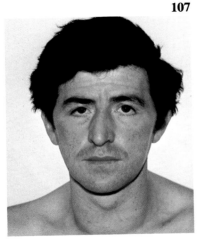 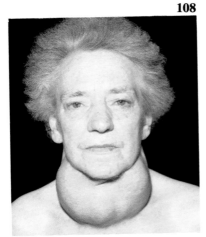

Classification of thyroid size

Various classifications of thyroid size are available but for routine clinical practice goitres are best defined as follows:

Small – thyroid palpable but not visible unless the neck is very thin.
Moderate – thyroid visible but not large (**107**).
Large – an obvious goitre which causes a definite increase in neck circumference (**108**).

Causes of goitre

The causes of goitre are virtually the same as those for hypothyroidism; most goitres represent an attempt to compensate for decreased circulating levels of thyroid hormones. **109** shows typical scan of a nodular goitre.

Prevalence of goitre

The prevalence of goitre varies in different parts of the world: in severely iodine-deficient areas endemic goitre may be seen in more than 90 per cent of the population.

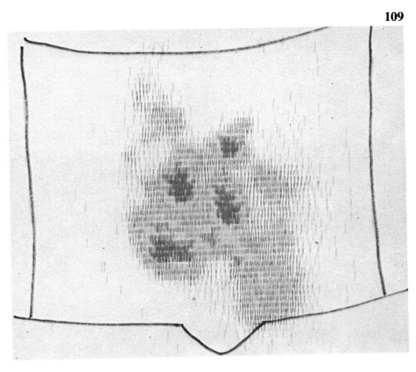

Clinical features of the different types of goitre

Types of goitre

The common types of goitre include the following:
1 Simple non-toxic goitre
2 Endemic goitre
3 Autoimmune thyroid disease
4 Thyroid nodules and neoplasms
5 Drug-induced goitre
6 Dyshormonogenesis
7 Ectopic goitre

Simple non-toxic goitre

The term 'simple goitre' can be used to describe those cases of thyroid enlargement where no detectable disturbance of thyroid function is present, and where no evident pathological explanation is available. Most goitres in the UK fall into this category, and treatment is rarely required unless there are pressure effects or a suspicion of malignancy. In younger age groups the thyroid is diffusely enlarged, whereas in older patients nodules may be visible as well as palpable – **109** shows a typical scan of a nodular goitre.

Degenerative changes with calcification may be evident on X-ray (see **110**); X-rays of the root of the neck may also show narrowing and displacement of the trachea or retrosternal extension (**111**). A palpable and sometimes visible pyramidal lobe extending upwards from the isthmus of the thyroid indicates some process causing generalised enlargement of the thyroid. Hyperthyroidism may develop in patients with long-standing nodular goitres, particularly after iodide administration.

110

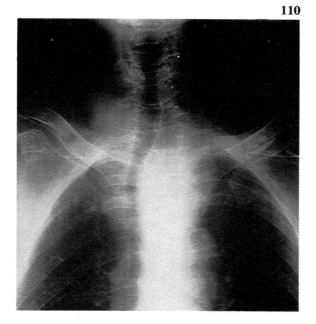

111

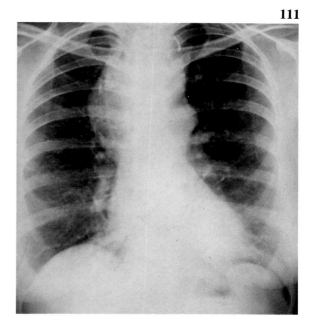

Drug-induced goitre

These show the sex ratio of the underlying disease rather than the usual female preponderance of most varieties of goitre. Hypothyroidism may accompany thyroid enlargement. Both are responsive to drug withdrawal and/or thyroid hormone administration (**73**).

Dyshormonogenesis

Goitres resulting from enzyme defects are uncommon except in children and are often familial. Thyroid disease is frequently associated with mental retardation, not necessarily due to thyroid hormone deficiency. Defects in the organification of iodine may be accompanied by deaf mutism. Certain defects may be associated with calcification visible on X-ray of the neck (**124**).

124

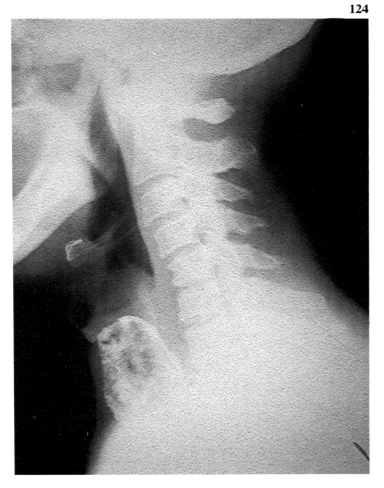

Ectopic goitre

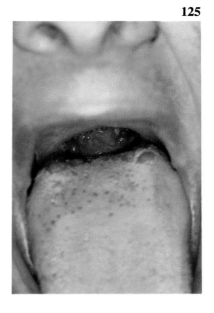

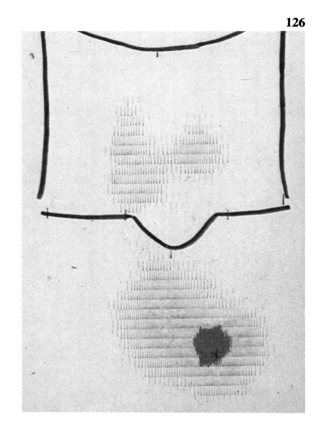

Ectopic thyroid tissue may be found anywhere on the path of descent of the thyroid from the root of the tongue (**125**) where it may cause dysphagia, to just above the thyroid isthmus or as far down as the mediastinum.

126 shows a scan of an ectopic thyroid in the upper mediastinum.

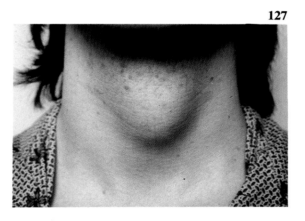

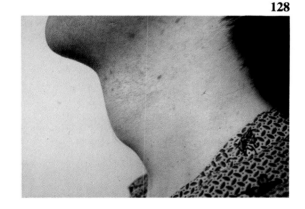

A thyroglossal cyst lies in the front of the larynx (**127** and **128**) and should be distinguished from an ectopic thyroid in this position associated with absence of thyroid tissue in the normal position.

Inadequate function of an impalpable ectopic thyroid (recognisable only on scanning) is a common cause of neonatal hypothyroidism.

4: Adrenal

Adrenal cortex

Introduction

The adrenal cortex secretes three groups of steroids, which are classified by their biological actions.

1 The glucocorticoids have major effects on glucose and protein metabolism, and a number of other metabolic actions. The most important glucocorticoids are cortisol, cortisone and corticosterone. Cortisol is the most potent glucocorticoid in man. Cortisone and 11-dehydrocorticosterone do not have intrinsic metabolic activity, but are active after conversion to cortisol and corticosterone. Glucocorticoid secretion is controlled by ACTH.

2 The mineralocorticoids are steroids which have a major effect on electrolyte transport by epithelial cells leading to sodium conservation and potassium loss. The most potent of these is aldosterone, but 11-deoxycorticosterone (DOC), 18-hydroxy–DOC, corticosterone, and cortisol all have some mineralocorticoid activity. Aldosterone secretion is regulated by the renin-angiotensin system.

3 The sex steroids (androgens and oestrogens) are secreted in small amounts under normal conditions. Excess production may, however, cause significant clinical problems.

Clinical features of adrenocortical disease

Cushing's syndrome

'Cushing's syndrome' is the term used to describe those clinical disorders resulting from an excess of circulating glucocorticoid. The term 'Cushing's disease' is used to describe patients in whom the syndrome results from an increase in pituitary ACTH production. This is the commonest cause of spontaneous Cushing's syndrome.

Causes of Cushing's syndrome

ACTH dependent	ACTH independent
Hypothalamic-pituitary dependent (Cushing's disease)	Adrenal adenoma
Ectopic ACTH syndrome	Adrenal carcinoma
ACTH therapy	Glucocorticoid therapy

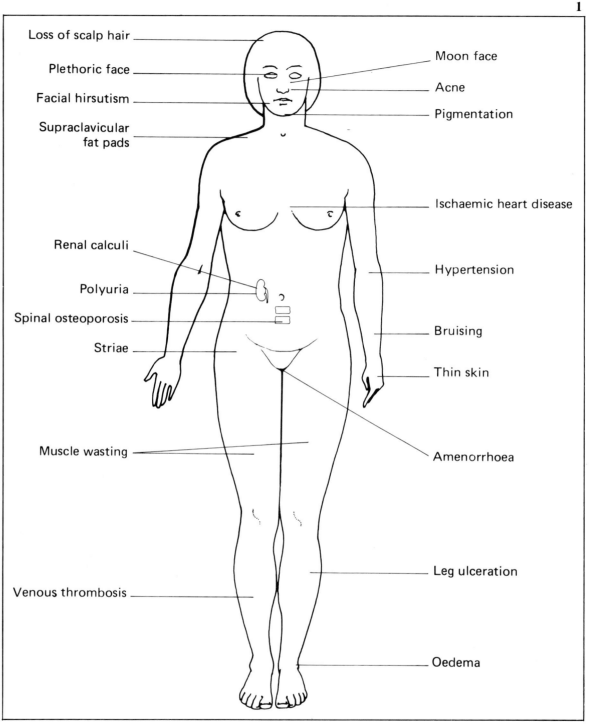

Loss of scalp hair

Plethoric face

Facial hirsutism

Supraclavicular
fat pads

Moon face

Acne

Pigmentation

Ischaemic heart disease

Renal calculi

Polyuria

Spinal osteoporosis

Striae

Hypertension

Bruising

Thin skin

Muscle wasting

Amenorrhoea

Venous thrombosis

Leg ulceration

Oedema

Cushing's syndrome

The common modes of presentation are obesity,
hirsutism, hypertension and symptoms related to
premature spinal osteoporosis. The diagnosis is
frequently suggested by the characteristic appearance of the patient (**1**).

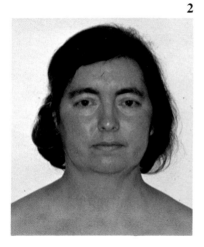

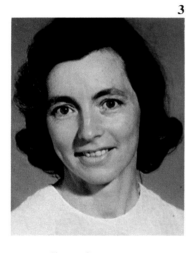

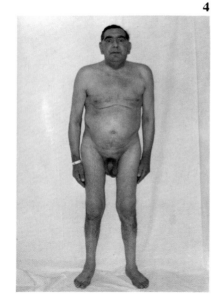

The most striking facial features are rounding of the face, plethora, hirsutism, loss of scalp hair, acne and pigmentation (2).

The facial appearance after treatment will revert to normal (3 same patient as in 2).

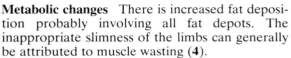

Metabolic changes There is increased fat deposition probably involving all fat depots. The inappropriate slimness of the limbs can generally be attributed to muscle wasting (4).

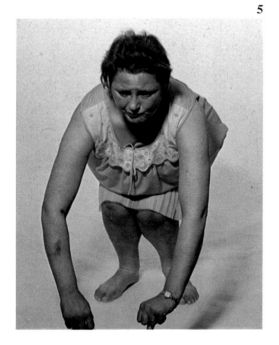

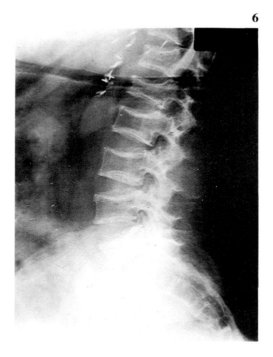

Muscle catabolism is increased leading to wasting and weakness (which may be increased by hypokalaemia). The weakness is generally most prominent in the proximal muscles; this can be demonstrated by asking the patient to rise from a crouched position without aid (5).

Increased protein catabolism may lead to osteoporosis with loss of height and pathological fractures (6).

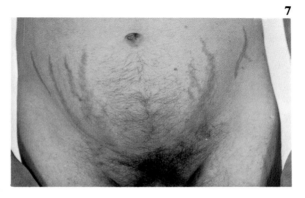

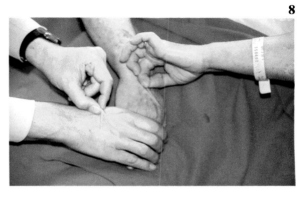

Characteristic thinning of the skin is due to protein loss and leads to the formation of purple striae

(7). Skin thickness can be assessed by raising a fold on the back of the patient's hand (8).

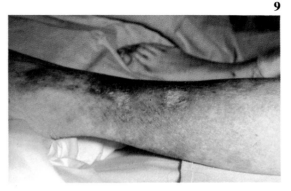

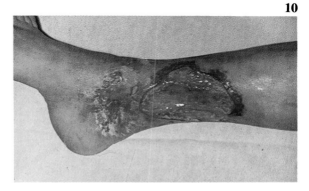

The fragility of vessel walls is increased leading to bruising (9).

The tissues in Cushing's syndrome generally have a reduced tensile strength as a result of increased protein catabolism and thus wound-healing is poor; spontaneous ulceration is not uncommon (10).

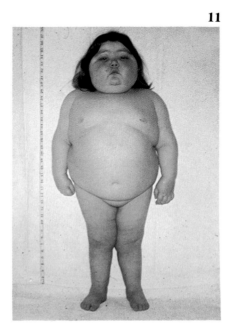

Growth retardation is seen in children and adolescents with Cushing's syndrome (11).

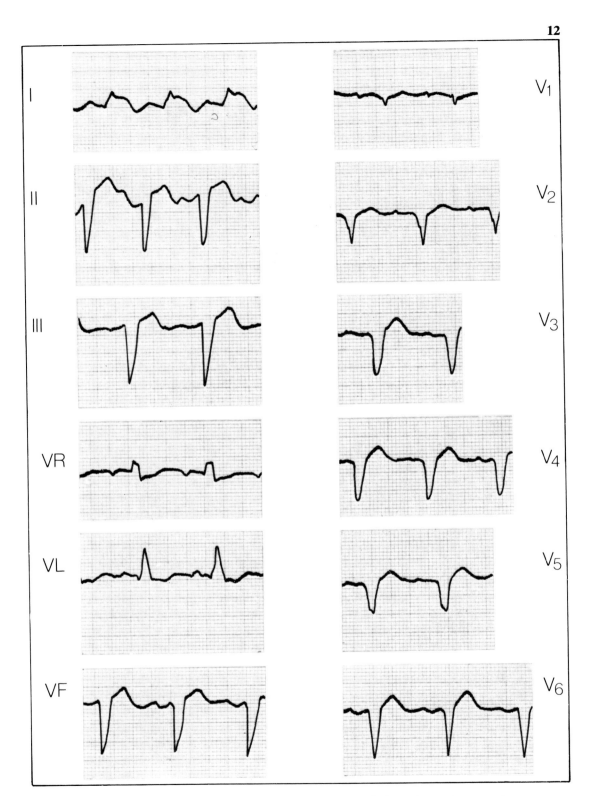

The cardiovascular system Hypertension is common and there is an increased incidence of ischaemic heart disease (**12**).

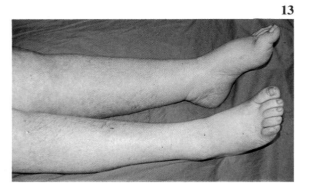

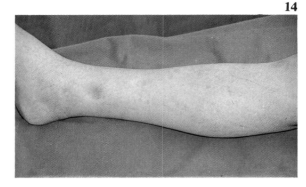

An increased risk of venous thrombosis is present (13).

Effects on water and electrolyte metabolism The glucocorticoids if present in excess lead to sodium retention, potassium loss and an increased free water clearance. The sodium retention may lead to oedema (14) and contribute to the hypertension.

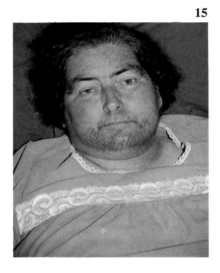

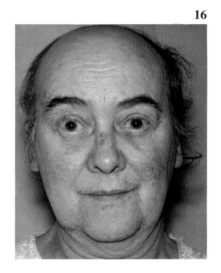

Abnormal androgen production Generally there is only a minor increase in androgen production in Cushing's disease. Amenorrhoea is almost invariable, hirsutism (15) and acne are common, but major degrees of virilisation are rare. 16 shows extensive male pattern balding in a female with Cushing's disease.

17

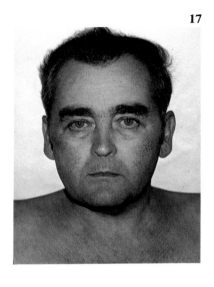

Increased ACTH production
ACTH is a pigmentary hormone and an increase in skin pigmentation is seen in some patients (**17**). The pigmentation is most marked in areas exposed to friction and in scars (**18**). The diagnosis is confirmed by demonstrating hypercortisolism and a moderate elevation of ACTH.

18

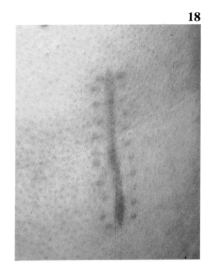

Post-adrenalectomy syndrome (Nelson's syndrome) Bilateral adrenalectomy for Cushing's disease is followed by the post-adrenalectomy syndrome in a proportion of patients. Expansion of the pituitary fossa and hyperpigmentation (**19**) may be present and, rarely, cranial nerve palsies.

19

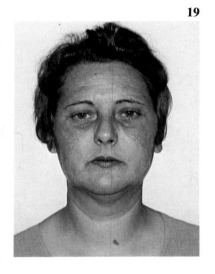

Ectopic ACTH syndrome Cushing's syndrome as a result of ectopic ACTH production generally follows a rapidly progressive clinical course. The typical facial appearance of the syndrome is often not apparent (**20**). The metabolic changes are severe reflecting the very high cortisol levels in this condition, leading to a major degree of muscle weakness and oedema.

20

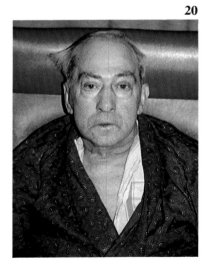

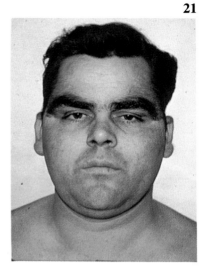

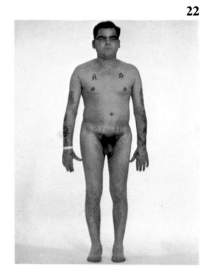

Severe pigmentation is common because of the very high levels of ACTH (**21** and **22**).

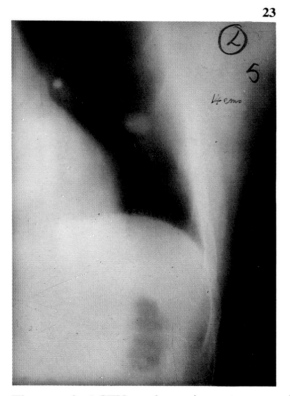

The ectopic ACTH syndrome is most commonly associated with bronchial carcinoma (**23**) and is, therefore, seen most frequently in males.

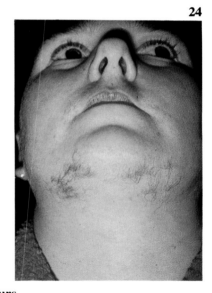

Adrenal tumours

Cushing's syndrome caused by an adrenal tumour frequently cannot be distinguished on clinical grounds from hypothalamic-pituitary dependent disease. A major degree of androgen overproduction is seen in some patients leading to a marked degree of virilisation (**24**).

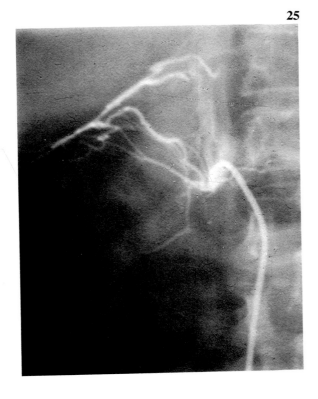

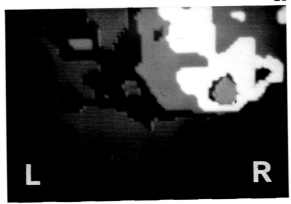

26

The adrenal tumour may be palpable and liver enlargement may be seen. The tumour may be identified by venography (**25**) angiography, labelled cholesterol scan (**26**), or selective venous sampling.

Primary aldosteronism

Primary aldosteronism may result from an adrenal tumour or hyperplasia of the zona glomerulosa. The characteristic biochemical features are hypernatraemia, hypokalaemia and suppression of renin production. Sodium retention leads to an increase in extracellular fluid volume (although oedema is rare) and hypertension.

Potassium loss leads to muscle weakness which may be sufficiently severe to cause periodic paralysis and impaired carbohydrate tolerance (**27**).

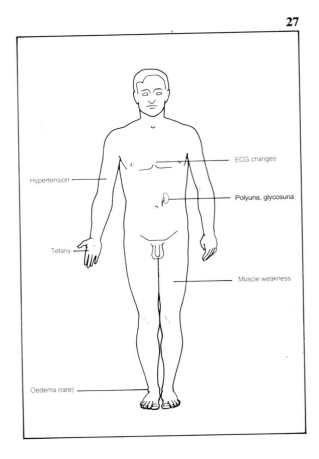

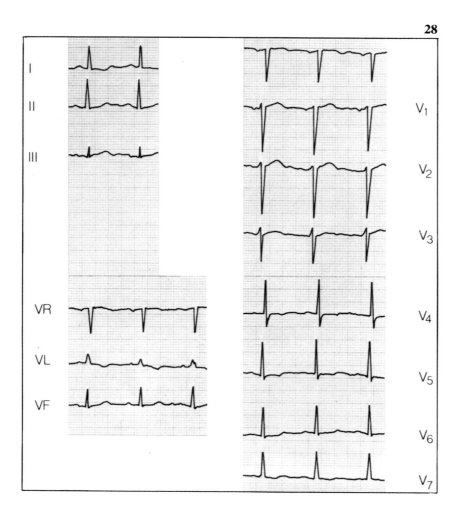

27

28

Cardiac abnormalities are common and include ST-T depression, U waves and ventricular premature contractions (**28**); hypokalaemic alkalosis may lead to tetany.

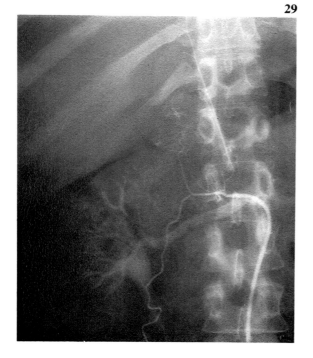

29

Hypokalaemic renal damage can give rise to polyuria and secondary polydipsia.

The tumour is generally small but may be demonstrated by iodocholesterol scan, aortography (**29**) or venography.

Hypoadrenalism

Chronic adrenocortical failure (**30**) (Addison's disease) is generally caused by an autoimmune process ('idiopathic Addison's disease') or by tuberculous destruction of the glands. Acute failure most commonly results from withdrawal of suppressive doses of steroids, surgical removal of the glands, or stress in patients with chronic failure, but may occasionally be precipitated by haemorrhage into the glands (Waterhouse–Friederichsen syndrome or anticoagulant therapy).

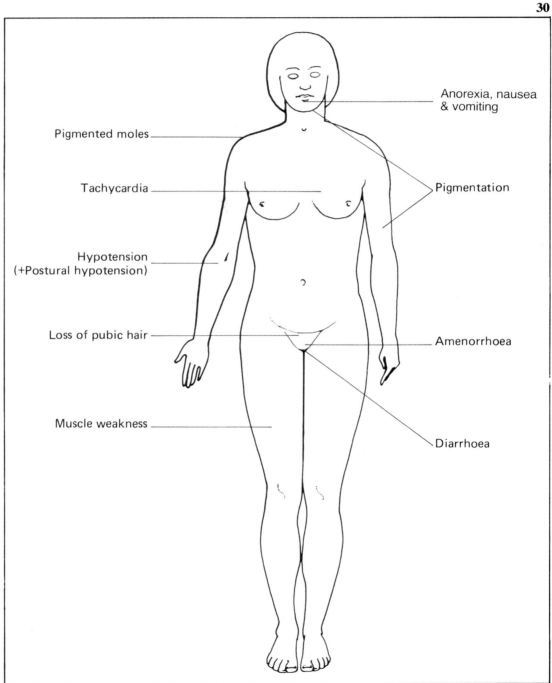

30

Pigmented moles

Tachycardia

Hypotension
(+Postural hypotension)

Loss of pubic hair

Muscle weakness

Anorexia, nausea
& vomiting

Pigmentation

Amenorrhoea

Diarrhoea

31

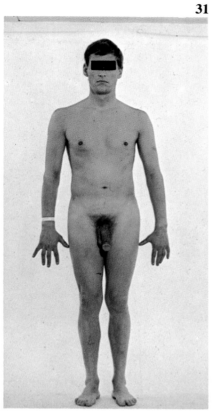

Glucocorticoid deficiency The major clinical manifestations are tiredness, weight loss, gastro-intestinal disturbance, hypoglycaemia and depression (**31**).

32

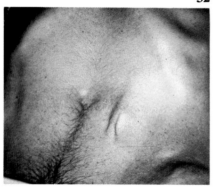

Mineralocorticoid deficiency Dehydration, hypotension and cramps are common. Reduced skin turgor (**32**) is evident in many patients.

33

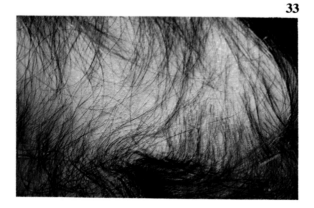

Androgen deficiency This may lead to hair loss in the female. **33** shows scalp hair loss.

Excess ACTH production will lead to increased pigmentation 34 shows a patient with Addison's disease on right photographed with her healthy identical twin sister.

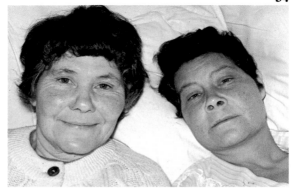

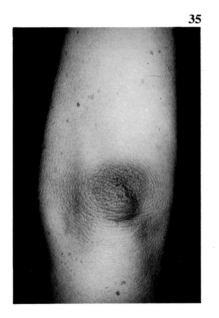

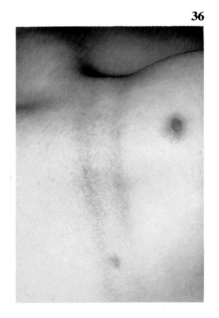

This is generally most marked in the skin creases and at areas of friction. 35 shows pigmentation over the elbow and 36 under an area of friction from a brassiere strap, and on the buccal mucosa (37).

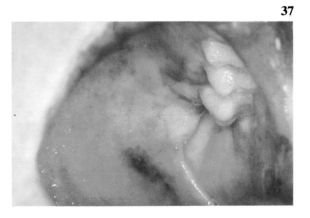

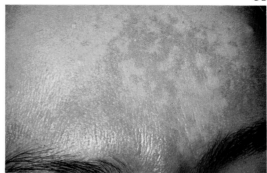

38

The pigmentation of melanosis or chloasma (**38**) may occasionally be confused with the pigmentation of hypoadrenalism.

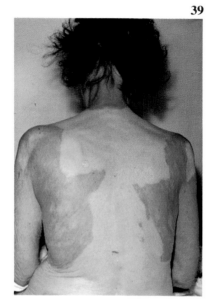

39

Associated features Vitiligo (a skin marker of organ-specific autoimmune disease) may be seen and provides a striking contrast to the hyper-pigmentation seen in other areas (**39**).

There is an association with other organ-specific autoimmune disorders (autoimmune thyroid disease, primary hypoparathyroidism, pernicious anaemia, premature ovarian failure).

Congenital adrenal hyperplasia

The synthesis of the adrenal steroids is dependent upon a number of enzymatically regulated stages. Congenital deficiency of any of these stages results in the under-production of some adrenal steroids and overproduction of others as biosynthesis is diverted down alternative metabolic pathways.

Six identifiable varieties of congenital adrenal hyperplasia exist – each attributable to a specific enzyme deficiency:

1   20-hydroxylase (cholesterol desmolase) deficiency
2   3 ß-hydroxysteroid deficiency
3   17-hydroxylase deficiency
4   21-hydroxylase deficiency
5   11 ß-hydroxylase deficiency
6   18-hydroxysteroid dehydrogenase deficiency

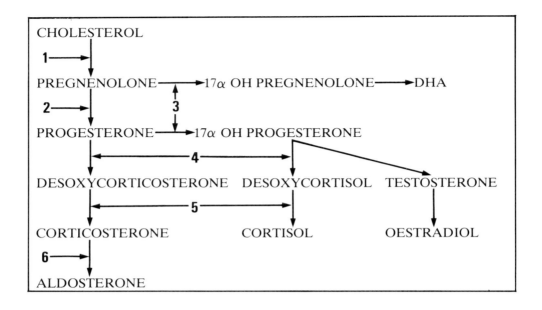

20-hydroxylase deficiency and 3 ß-hydroxysteroid deficiency Patients with these disorders manifest severe glucocorticoid and mineralocorticoid deficiency from birth and require urgent replacement therapy. Problems of sexual differentiation occur because these infants are phenotypically female whether the genotype is XX or XY (see page 113). Delayed puberty presents clinical problems at a later age.

17-hydroxylase deficiency This condition is characterised by hypertension caused by excessive production of desoxycorticosterone and corticosterone. Deficient androgen production may lead to problems of sexual differentiation or delayed puberty, as in patients with 20-hydroxylase or 3 ß-hydroxysteroid deficiency.

21-hydroxylase deficiency This is the commonest variety of congenital adrenal hyperplasia and is associated with pseudoprecocious puberty in the male and virilisation in the female. Occasionally mineralocorticoid deficiency may be severe and lead to hypotension and hyperkalaemia.

11 ß-hydroxylase deficiency This deficiency is characterised by pseudoprecocious puberty in the male and virilisation in the female, in association with systemic hypertension (secondary to overproduction of desoxycorticosterone).

18-hydroxysteroid dehydrogenase deficiency Deficiency of this enzyme leads to pure aldosterone deficiency causing hyperkalaemia, hyponatraemia and hypotension.

Clinical features of disease of the adrenal medulla – phaeochromocytoma

The catecholamines are important neurotransmitters and are secreted by tissues of neural crest origin. The major amines are dopamine, noradrenaline (norepinephrine) and adrenaline (epinephrine). The adrenal medullae are minor sources of catecholamines.

Phaeochromocytoma is usually a benign tumour secreting catecholamines. Approximately 90 per cent are found in the adrenal medullae, the remainder being associated with other sympathetic tissue. The tumours may be multiple.

The characteristic clinical features (**40**) are intermittent or sustained hypertension (**41**) paroxysmal attacks with blanching, palpitations, tachycardia, and sweating. Tremulousness, anxiety and disturbance of sleep are common additional manifestations.

PHAEOCHROMOCYTOMA
(and associated conditions)

Sweating

Facial haemangioma

Epiloia

Medullary
carcinoma of thyroid

Cafe au lait spots &
neurofibromata

Tachycardia and
palpitations

Hypertension

Tremor

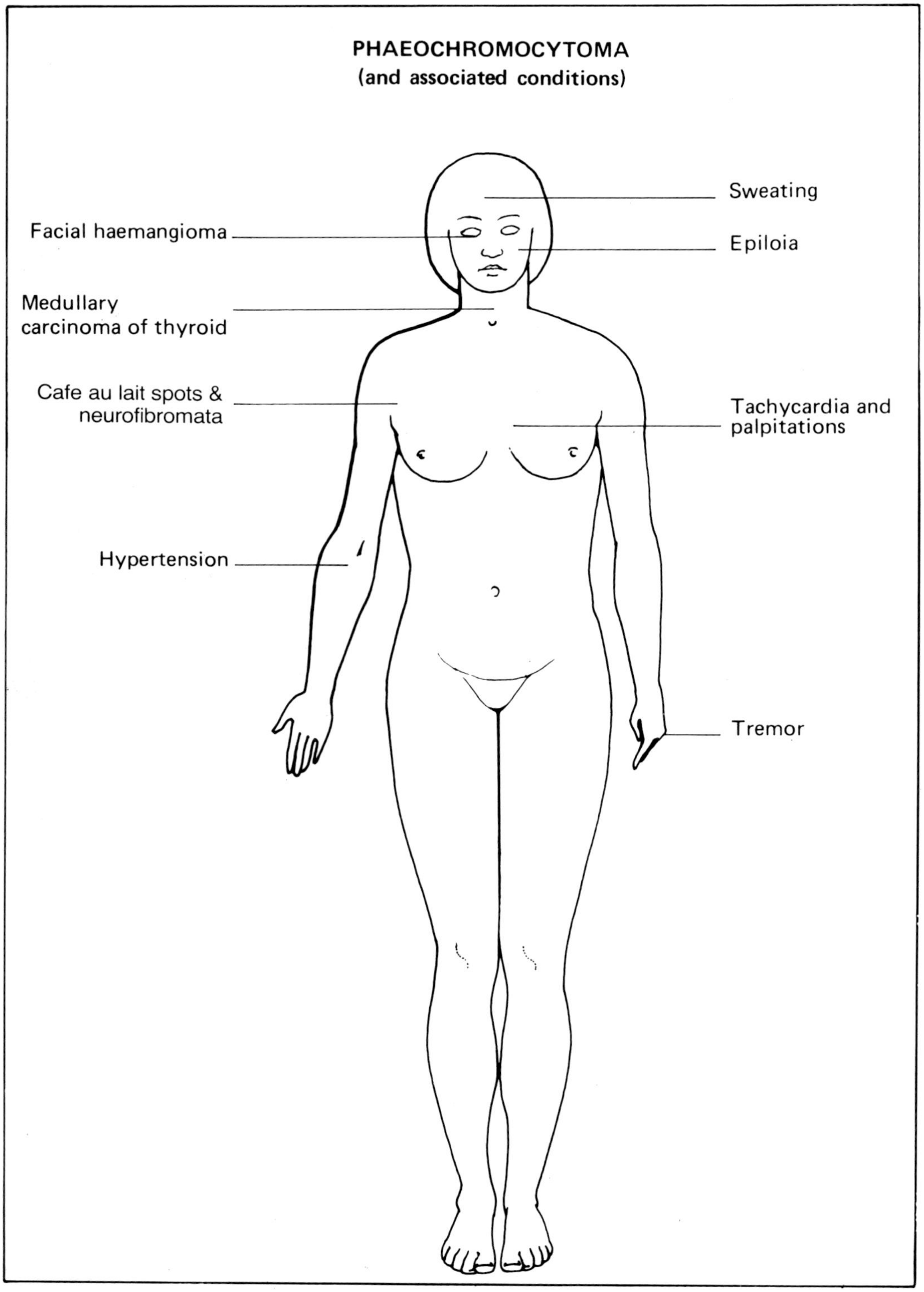

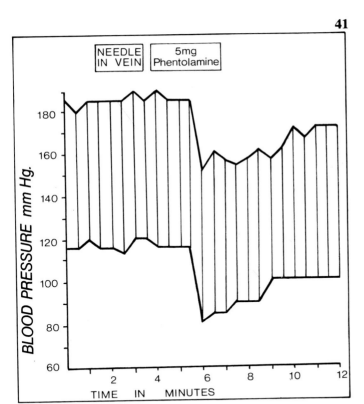

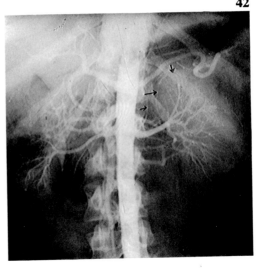

Phaeochromocytomas can be localised by aortography (**42**), venography or calcification on X-ray.

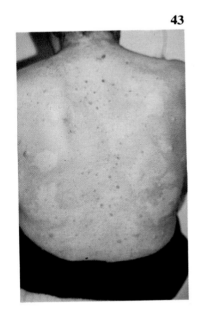

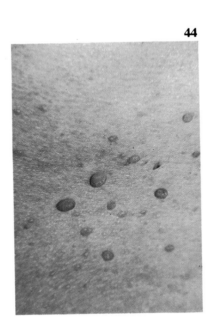

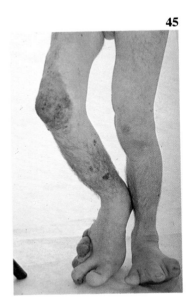

There is an association between phaeochromocytoma and the neuroectodermal diseases, of which neurofibromatosis is the most frequent (**43** and **44**). An association with Lindau's disease (neural haemangiomata, visceral cysts and hypernephroma) is also seen (**45**).

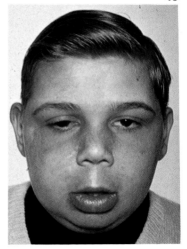

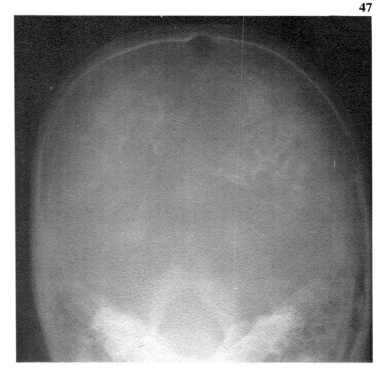

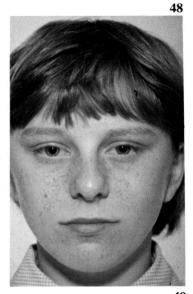

There is also an association with Sturge–Weber disease (encephalofacial angiomatosis) (**46** and **47** show facial appearance and typical gyral calcification) and tuberose sclerosis. (**48** shows adenoma sebaceum.)

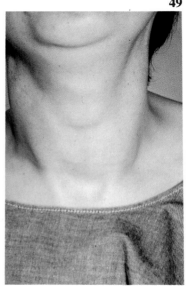

There is also an association between phaeochromocytoma and the familial form of medullary carcinoma of the thyroid – 'Sipple's syndrome' (**49**).

Cryptorchidism

Undescended testes are common at birth (about 10 per cent of male births) but normal descent will occur in most patients. The testes remain in the abdomen or inguinal canal in true cryptorchidism; a high proportion show abnormalities of development. A significant risk of malignancy exists in cryptorchidism. **12** shows an empty scrotal sac in cryptorchidism.

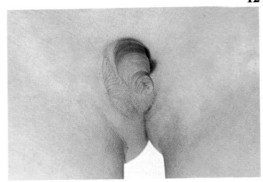

True cryptorchidism must be distinguished from pseudocryptorchidism or retractile testes, which can be massaged into the scrotum (**13**). Reduced fertility and impaired development of secondary sexual characteristics are common in cryptorchidism.

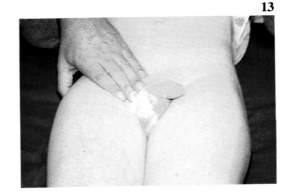

Testicular agenesis (anorchia)

Patients with testicular agenesis commonly have a male phenotype; thus testicular failure must have occurred after the seventh to fourteenth week of foetal life, because failure before this age will lead to a female phenotype. These patients generally have small palpable masses in the scrotum, the vas deferens is palpable, and they go through normal development up to the time of puberty. The condition may be familial. **14** shows testicular agenesis; the patient had received a small dose of androgens.

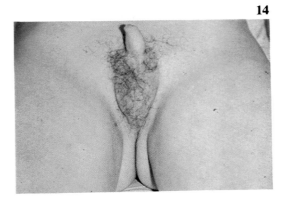

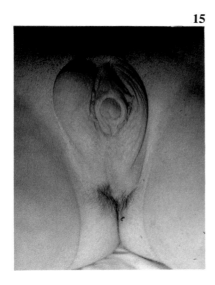

Reifenstein's syndrome This syndrome is the association of hypospadias, postpubertal testicular atrophy affecting spermatogenesis and endocrine function. The scrotum is bifid (**15**).

Eunuchoidism and gynaecomastia complete the clinical picture. The syndrome is limited to males and is inherited either as an X-linked recessive or a male-limited autosomal dominant.

Congenital adrenal hyperplasia

21-hydroxylase deficiency The severity of the abnormalities may vary considerably. The female, if severely affected, may show marked virilisation with clitoral hypertrophy and partial fusion of labioscrotal folds. **16** shows a severely affected child with a major degree of labioscrotal fusion. The patient may be mistaken for a male with cryptorchidism and hypospadias. Milder forms may be unrecognised. Clitoral hypertrophy may be minor and the patients correctly identified as female (**17**). The condition is frequently unrecognised in the male unless very severe and associated with salt-wasting and hypotension.

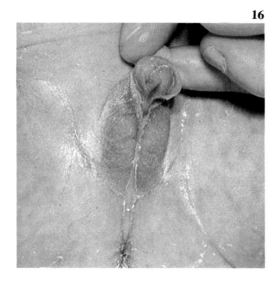

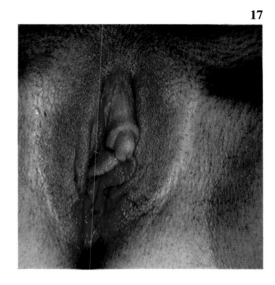

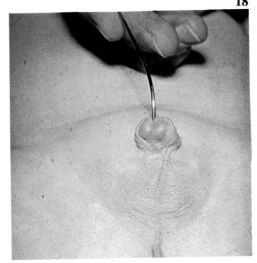

11 ß-hydroxylase deficiency The clinical features of this syndrome resemble those of the 21 hydroxylase deficiency with respect to sexual development (**18**), but clinically 11ß-hydroxylase deficiency can be distinguished by the presence of hypertension. This syndrome is much less common than 21-hydroxylase deficiency.

Disorders in phenotypic females

Chromosomal disorders

The only important disorder in this category is Turner's syndrome and its variants. This is a chromosomally determined disorder where complete ovarian agenesis is present with deletion of one X chromosome (karyotype 45 XO). Incomplete forms may be seen in patients with mosaicism (XO/XX, XO/XXX, XO/XX/XXX), in which case the patient may be chromatin positive. The features are shown in **19**.

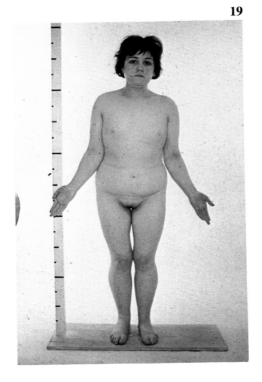

Turner's syndrome is generally suspected on clinical grounds by the association of primary amenorrhoea, sexual immaturity, shortness of stature and the characteristic physical stigmata which include webbing of the neck (about 40 per cent of patients), and increased carrying angle at the elbow (cubitus valgus). The chest tends to be square and the nipples are small and widely spaced (**19**).

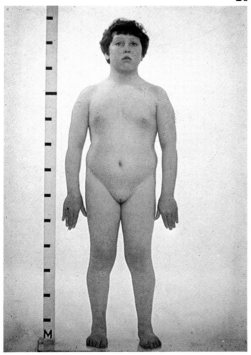

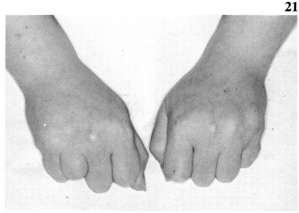

21

The hands may show puffiness of the dorsum and a short fourth metacarpal, which is demonstrated by asking the patient to make a fist (**21**). Hypoplasia of the nails is occasionally seen.

Other anomalies which may be seen include lymphoedema of the feet and hands, an excess of pigmented naevi, and a tendency to keloid formation.

Examination of the face may reveal epicanthal folds, micrognathia, a fish-like mouth, deformed or low-set ears (**20**) and/or a low hair line.

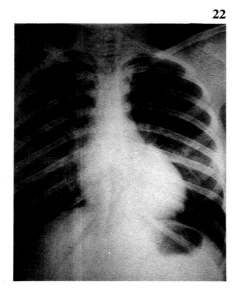

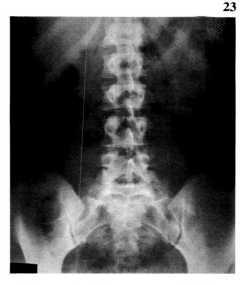

A number of radiological findings may be seen including effusions into serous cavities and the features of coarctation of the aorta (**22**). Pyelography may reveal a horseshoe kidney or anomalies of the renal pelvis or ureters; (**23** shows (R) renal agenesis) rounding of the medial femoral condyle and squaring of the lateral tibial condyle with a spur may be seen.

Turner's syndrome may be associated with hypo-thyroidism or diabetes mellitus.

The diagnosis can be confirmed by the typical 45 XO chromosome picture and the absence of Barr bodies (**24, 25**).

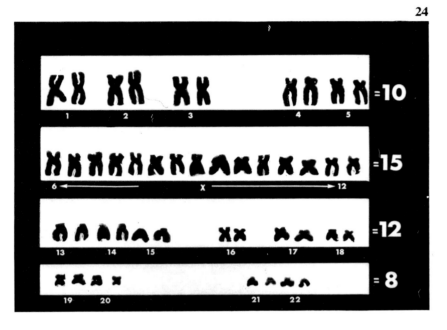

24

Turner's syndrome

chromatin negative

Karyotype	Sex chromosomes
45 X O	
Mosaic 45 XO/46 XY	
Mosaic 45 XO/46 XF	

F = small fragment of X or Y

It may be a small ring

Pure gonadal dysgenesis

26

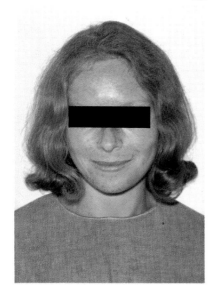

27

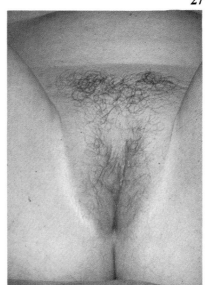

28

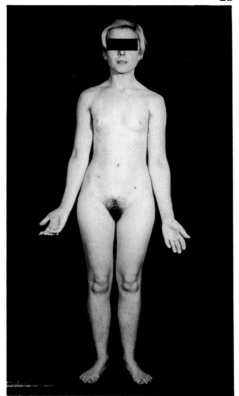

Pure gonadal dysgenesis may be associated with XX or XY karyotype. The patients are phenotypically female (**26**) and generally of normal or above average height. They present sexual infantilism and primary amenorrhoea at the time of puberty. **27** shows sexual infantilism in a 46XX adult with gonadal dysgenesis; **28** shows a 46XY adult with gonadal dysgenesis.

Incomplete forms may be seen and are associated with varying degrees of differentiation of the external genitalia and gonads. A high risk of tumour formation is present in dysgenetic gonads, particularly in the XY form. Gonadal calcification may be seen on X-ray.

Congenital adrenal hyperplasia

(These defects may affect the gonads as well as the adrenals.)

20-hydroxylase (cholesterol desmolase) deficiency
Infants with this anomaly have female external genitalia (whether the karyotype is XX or XY).

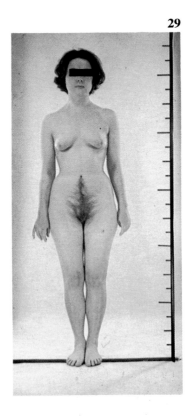

29

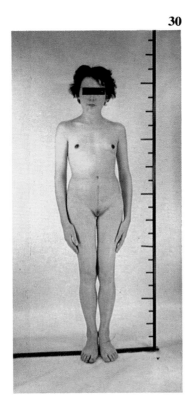

30

3 ß-hydroxysteroid dehydrogenase deficiency Most reported cases have died in infancy, but patients with partial defects survive causing male pseudohermaphroditism in the male and partial masculinisation in the female (**29**).

17-hydroxylase deficiency This disorder is characterised by a failure to synthesise and secrete androgens or oestrogens. Sexual infantilism in a phenotypic female in association with hypertension is the characteristic finding in this group (**30**).

Testicular feminisation

Complete testicular feminisation This is a highly distinctive inherited disorder in which half of the genotypic males in an affected family are phenotypically female. There is a tissue resistance to androgens and thus wolffian-duct structures are poorly (although partially) developed. Complete involution of the mullerian ducts is present, since 'mullerian inhibiting substance' is produced normally.

31

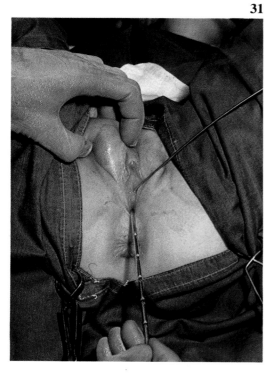

32

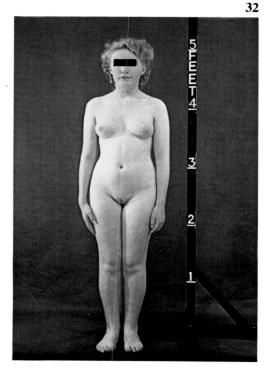

The external genitalia are female. The 'vagina' is shallow and ends in a blind pouch. The testes are found in the labia majora (**31**), inguinal canals or intra-abdominally. The Leydig cells become hyperplastic at puberty and tend to form adenomata.

Female secondary sex characteristics develop during the second decade. Rounding of body contours with generally well-developed breasts is present. Feminisation probably occurs as a result of increased oestrogen levels, which are driven by relatively high gonadotrophins because of the insensitivity of the normal feedback mechanism to androgens. Sexual hair is scanty or absent (**32**).

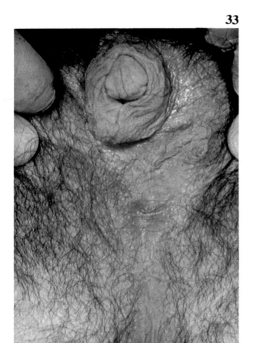

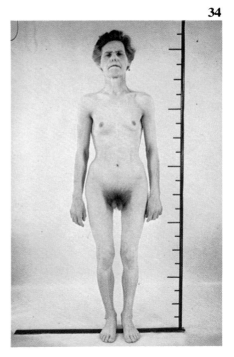

34

Incomplete testicular feminisation This is a variant of the above syndrome in which there is some phallic enlargement and partial labioscrotal fusion (**33**).

Breast development is less marked at puberty and hirsutism or partial virilisation may be evident (**34**).

Absent or anomalous genitalia

Absence or anomalous development of fallopian tubes, uterus and/or vagina may occur and congenital absence of the vagina may pose gender identification problems. These anomalies do not have an endocrine cause. They may be associated with congenital absence of one kidney. **35** shows a nephrogram on the left side only at aortography.

Intermediate phenotypes

A number of the conditions described above may have intermediate phenotypes, particularly chromosomal mosaics and some forms of congenital adrenal hyperplasia.

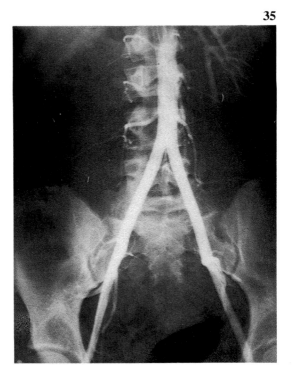

35

True hermaphroditism

The diagnosis of true hermaphroditism depends upon the finding of ovarian and testicular tissue in the same or different gonads. The external genitalia are variable, male and female forms are seen but the genitalia are ambiguous in most cases. Most patients, however, are reared as males because of the size of the phallus, although hypospadias is almost invariably present; there is variable fusion of the labioscrotal folds.

36

37

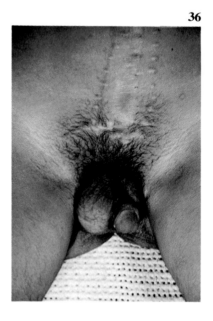

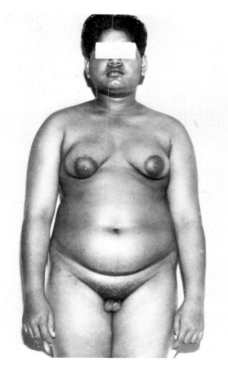

The gonads may be in the labioscrotal folds, the inguinal canal or the abdomen. The genital ducts are generally female in those patients with bilateral ovotestes, but in patients with an ovary on one side and testis on the other, the genital duct development generally follows the gonad on that side. **36** shows genitalia in true hermaphroditism.

Some breast development is present in about two-thirds of patients (**37**). Chromosomal examination reveals a 46XX constitution in about 45 per cent of patients, 46XY in about 20 per cent and mosaics in the remainder.

Errors of testosterone synthesis

Ambiguous genitalia may be seen in patients with 17, 20-desmolase deficiency or 17 ß-hydroxysteroid oxidoreductase deficiency. Both these conditions are very rare.

38

Disorders presenting as precocious puberty

Males

Precocious puberty in males is generally defined as the onset of pubertal changes before 10 years of age. This is an arbitrary but useful criterion.

True precocious puberty

Forty per cent of males with pubertal development before 10 years of age have no detectable organic disease. The diagnosis can only be made by exclusion of other causes of precocious puberty. Familial examples have been described. **38** shows genitalia in an 8-year-old boy with precocious puberty.

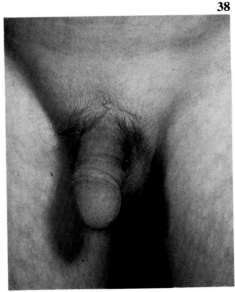

Congenital adrenal hyperplasia

21-hydroxylase deficiency and 11 ß-hydroxylase deficiency (v.s.) may lead to precocious puberty. The onset of pubertal changes occurs between 2 and 10 years of age, although testicular enlargement does not occur; the patients are not potentially fertile. There is a period of rapid linear growth, increased muscularity and the early appearance of pubic and axillary hair. Acne may be marked. The two causes may be distinguished clinically by the occurrence of hypertension in the latter.

39

Premature epiphyseal fusion is present and thus the 'final' height of affected subjects is reduced (**39**).

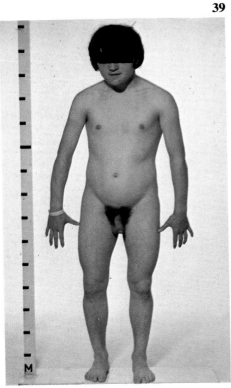

Rare causes

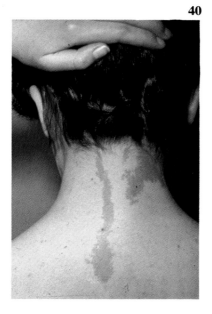

40

Precocious puberty may be associated with a number of cerebral tumours which affect the hypothalamus. The presence of hypothalamic disease may be suggested by changes in behaviour, sleep or feeding habit. The presence of a glioma may be suggested by the finding of neurofibromatosis (see page 101). A rare but well-documented association exists between hypothyroidism and sexual precocity, which may reflect hypothalamic disturbance. Precocious puberty is occasionally associated with polyostotic fibrous dysplasia (Albright's syndrome) (**40** shows the typical pigmentation) or with a hepatoblastoma.

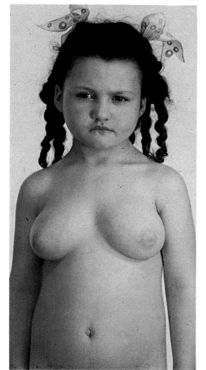

41

Females

Precocious puberty in females is generally defined as the onset of sexual maturation before 8 years of age.

True precocious puberty

Most girls (80 per cent) with pubertal development before 8 years of age have no detectable organic disease. **41** shows a 4-year-old girl with true precocious puberty.

Congenital adrenal hyperplasia

42

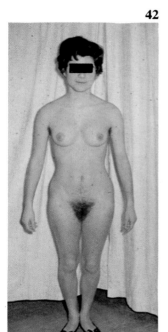

43

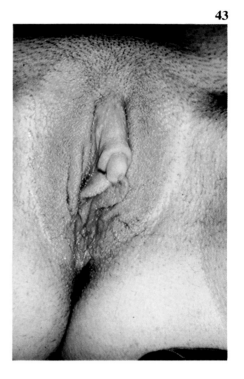

Females with 21-hydroxylase and 11 ß-hydroxylase deficiency may develop some features of sexual precocity with increased muscular development (**42**). Breast development may be poor because of the increased androgen production. Pubertal changes are associated with virilisation (**43**).

Rare causes

Precocious puberty in the female (as in the male) may rarely be associated with brain tumours, hypothyroidism or polyostotic fibrous dysplasia. Ovarian or adrenal tumours may be associated with sexual precocity in the female.

Disorders presenting as delayed puberty

Males

The onset of puberty in boys generally occurs between 10 and 16 years of age. The child or his parents will usually seek medical advice if sexual maturation has not occurred by the latter age.

Constitutional delay in puberty

The age of onset of puberty varies considerably but is partly determined by the age of onset of puberty of the parents. The diagnosis of constitutional delay of puberty can be made if full clinical examination, serum gonadotrophins and testosterone and radiological bone age are normal.

A variant is the syndrome of apparently small genitalia in fat boys. The reduction in genital size is apparent rather than real, for the penile shaft is buried in the suprapubic fat pad and is normal in size. The testes are also normal in size for a prepubertal boy. This condition (44) is frequently misdiagnosed as the very rare Fröhlich's syndrome due to a hypothalamic tumour.

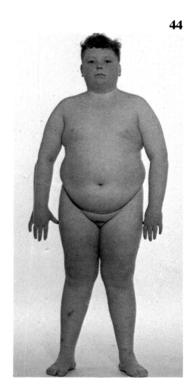

44

Organic causes of delay in puberty

True delay in puberty may occur as a result of hypothalamic or pituitary disease (see page 13) or primary testicular disease. Testicular disease causing delayed puberty most commonly occurs as a result of chromosomal disorders (see pages 104–106), other developmental anomalies (see pages 107–108) or other testicular disease (for example, orchitis, use of cytotoxic drugs).

If the patient does not receive androgen therapy secondary sexual characteristics do not develop, the skin remains fine, and fine wrinkling develops around the mouth (45).

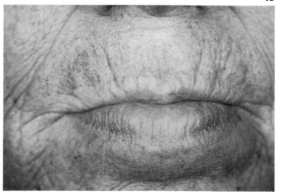

45

Females

The onset of puberty in girls generally occurs between the ages of 9 and 15 years of age. Menstruation generally starts between 10 and 17 years and may be irregular for one to two years before a more regular pattern develops.

Constitutional delay in puberty

Constitutional delay in puberty in the female (**46** and **47** both patients 18 years of age) as in the male, can only be identified after excluding hypothalamic, pituitary, ovarian or chromosomal disorders.

46

47

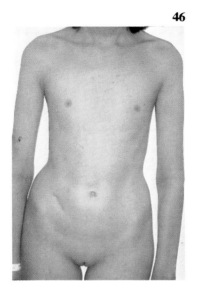
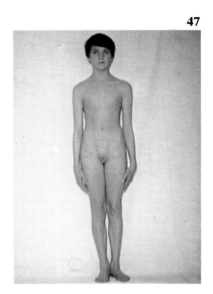

Organic causes of delay in puberty

True delay in puberty may occur as a result of hypothalamic or pituitary disease (see page 13), or disorders of sexual development (see pages 109–112). Prolonged primary amenorrhoea is associated with a failure to develop secondary sexual characteristics.

49

48 and **49** show a patient with Kallman's syndrome of hypogonadotrophic hypogonadism associated with anosmia.

48

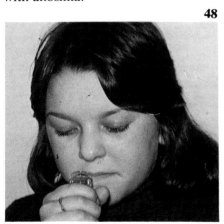

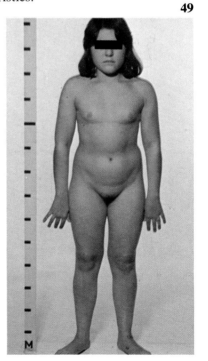

Disorders presenting as secondary amenorrhoea or infertility

Secondary amenorrhoea or infertility are common causes for referral to endocrine or gynaecological clinics. It is important to remember that pregnancy is the commonest cause of secondary amenorrhoea and that all contraceptive techniques are fallible, before extensive investigation is started.

Physiological secondary amenorrhoea

The commonest cause of secondary amenorrhoea, as stated previously, is caused by pregnancy. Periods of amenorrhoea may also be observed in the early years of menstruation, after parturition and also in the years just before the menopause.

'Functional' secondary amenorrhoea

Amenorrhea may accompany psychological or physical stress. Psychological illness or anxiety in young women may be accompanied by temporary cessation of periods. Physical illness or malnutrition can have a similar effect; secondary amenorrhoea is invariably present in anorexia nervosa (**50** and **51**).

50

51

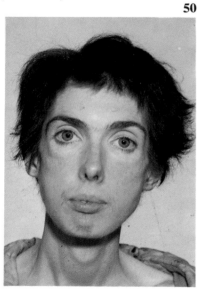

Hypothalamic-pituitary disease

Hypothalamic and/or pituitary disease is frequently accompanied by secondary amenorrhoea and infertility (see page 13). The presence of hyperprolactinaemia, with or without galactorrhoea (**52**), is common and may play a major part in the suppression of ovarian function. It is not always possible to identify a cause for the galactorrhoea, although a proportion of subjects with 'idiopathic' galactorrhoea will ultimately develop detectable pituitary tumours.

52

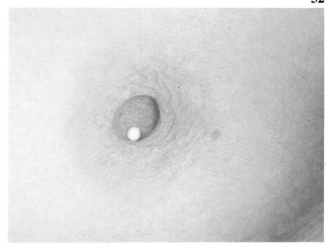

Ovarian disease

Premature ovarian failure Premature menopause is relatively common. It is often not possible to identify a cause, but it is thought in some patients to result from an autoimmune process. The condition may be associated with other autoimmune disorders, particularly Addison's disease. **53** shows Addison's disease. The symptoms and clinical features of ovarian failure are similar to those of the normal menopause.

53

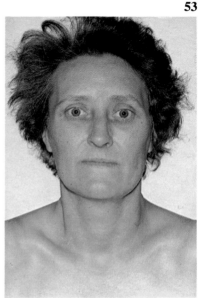

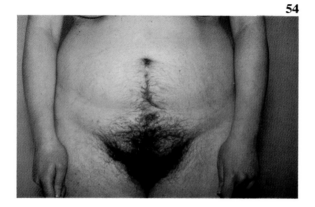

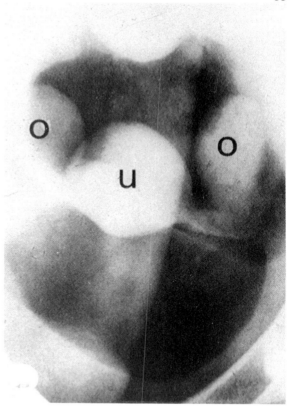

Polycystic ovary syndrome The major clinical features are obesity, amenorrhoea (or gross menstrual irregularity), hirsutism (**54**) and infertility. The ovaries are enlarged with a thickened capsule and contain multiple cysts. **55** shows ovarian enlargement (0) observed during gynaecography.

Ovarian hyperthecosis syndrome This is probably no more than a variant of the polycystic ovary syndrome. The clinical features of the two are indistinguishable, but the ovaries are relatively smaller and do not contain cysts; however, an excess of thecal cells is present in the ovarian stroma.

Masculinising ovarian tumours These tumours are rare. Amenorrhoea occurs early in the clinical course. Virilisation with coarsening of the skin, hirsutism, acne, breast atrophy, and clitoral hypertrophy develop with time. **56** and **57** show hirsutism and clitoral hypertrophy.

56

57

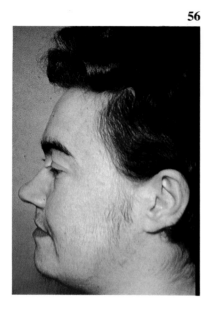

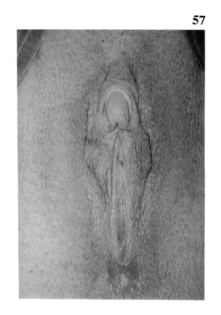

Other causes Secondary amenorrhoea and reduced fertility may also be seen in a number of other endocrine disorders (for example, Cushing's syndrome, hyperthyroidism), and serious organic disease, or after treatment with a number of drugs (for example, oral contraceptives, phenothiazines, tricyclic antidepressants and some antihypertensives). Simple obesity may also be associated with secondary amenorrhoea without any evident endocrine disorder.

Disorders presenting as hirsutism or virilism

Hirsutism cannot be defined objectively. The complaint of hirsutism by the patient is always an indication for physical examination; if the physician considers that the degree of hirsutism falls outside the wide limits of normality, then investigation may be necessary. There is considerable physiological variation between individuals, families and ethnic groups. Significant organic disease causing hirsutism (58) is almost invariably associated with amenorrhoea.

Virilisation describes the presence of some or all of the following features:

Temporal baldness
Deepening of the voice
Breast atrophy
Masculine habitus
Clitoral hypertrophy

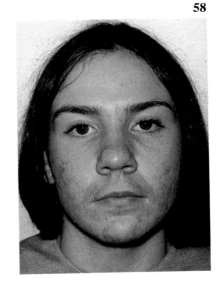

58

The causes of hirsutism and virilisation have been covered in other sections:

Adrenal   Cushing's syndrome (pages 85–93)
           Adrenal tumours (pages 92–93)
           Congenital adrenal hyperplasia
           (pages 98–99)

Ovarian   Polycystic ovary syndrome
           (page 124)
           Ovarian hyperthecosis syndrome
           (page 124)
           Masculinising tumours (page 124)

Drugs   Androgens
         Glucocorticoids
         Phenytoin

It is not possible to identify a cause of hirsutism which appears to fall outside the limits of normality in a proportion of patients.

6: Disorders of the breast

In the male the breast normally remains quiescent throughout life, apart from the physiological enlargement seen in most boys at puberty. In the female enlargement of the breast at puberty is followed by cyclical changes related to the menstrual cycle and secretory activity in response to pregnancy and suckling. Hormonal influences on the breast are complex and poorly understood; dominant effects are the result of oestrogens, progesterone, prolactin, human placental lactogen, and growth hormone while minor effects can be attributed to thyroid hormones and corticosteroids. The breast can only respond in a limited number of ways to pathological processes either by enlargement, atrophy or milk secretion.

Disorders of the male breast

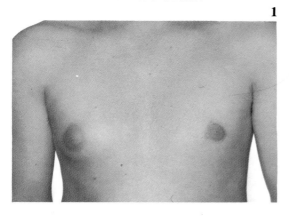

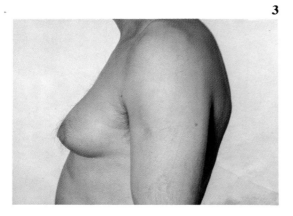

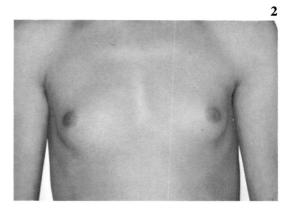

Enlargement of breast tissue occurs in most boys as an early event of puberty. Thus puberty gynaecomastia may be unilateral (**1**) or bilateral (**2**) and is only infrequently sufficiently prominent to cause embarrassment (**3**).

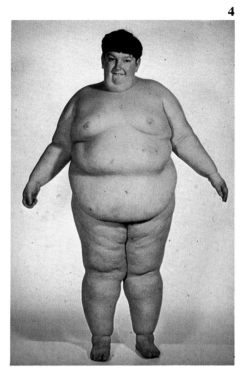

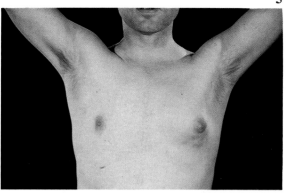

5

Puberty gynaecomastia should not be confused with the fatty swelling of the breast region seen in any obese male (4), in which it is not possible to palpate glandular tissue when the hand is applied firmly to the breast and pressed against the chest wall. An abscess may cause unilateral gynaecomastia; the condition usually follows local trauma in a patient with pre-existing gynaecomastia (5).

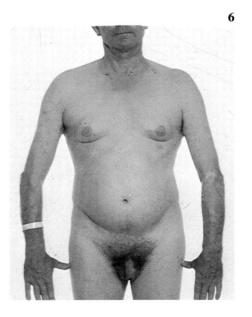

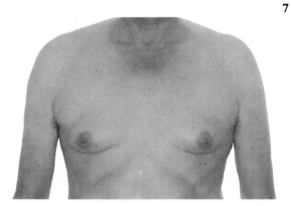

Oestrogen ingestion or production by tumours can cause gynaecomastia. 6 and 7 show breast enlargement in a 50-year-old man with an oestrogen-secreting adrenocortical carcinoma.

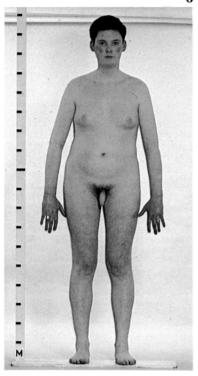

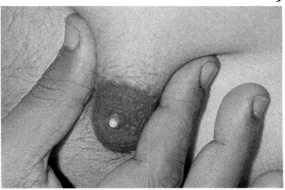

Secretion from the male breast can occur in a variety of conditions. Brown secretion may be seen in men treated with anabolic steroids for aplastic anaemia. True galactorrhoea in men (9) can result from any of the conditions causing this in females, particularly hyperprolactinaemic states resulting from drugs or hypothalamic pituitary disease, or from the lactogenic action of growth hormone in acromegaly (see Chapter 1).

When gynaecomastia is marked the possibility of Klinefelter's syndrome should be considered (8), but the small firm pea-sized testes associated with this condition are usually easily differentiated from the larger testes of a boy entering puberty.

Disorders of the female breast

These disorders may be congenital or acquired. Congenital absence of breast tissue is usually associated with maldevelopment of the pectoralis major (10), but can also indicate some chromosomal anomaly. 11 shows lack of breast development in a 17-year-old phenotypic female with gonadal dysgenesis and a 46XY karyotype. In Turner's syndrome the nipples are poorly developed and widely spaced and the breasts usually atrophic (12).

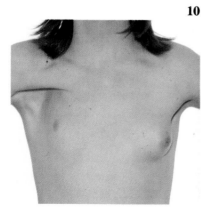
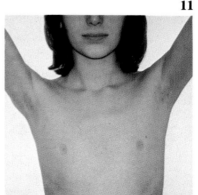
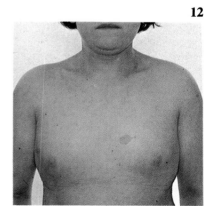

10

13

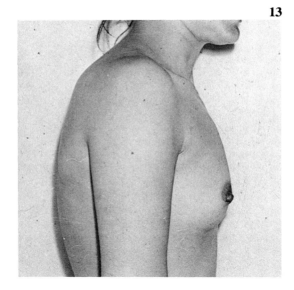

14

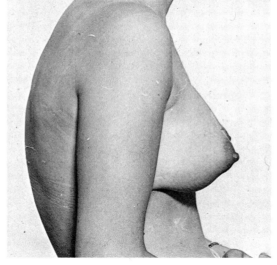

15

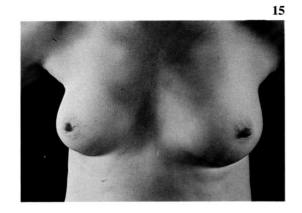

Small breasts usually represent the lower end of the normal range and do not preclude normal suckling. Secondary atrophy of the breasts may occur without cause or may follow a period of weight loss. The improvement in appearance produced by Silastic implants is usually mirrored by a dramatic psychological improvement. **13** and **14** show breast atrophy and the result after Silastic implant. Asymmetrical breasts are common but this is only rarely so marked as to cause concern (**15**).

Large breasts may occur as a primary phenomenon or may develop in adult life without any obvious cause. **16** and **17** show a patient with large breasts before and after plastic surgery. Obesity is usually accompanied by deposition of fat in the breasts which remits with weight reduction.

16

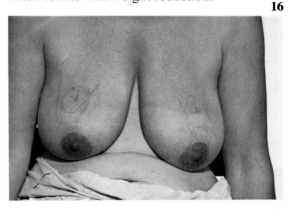

17

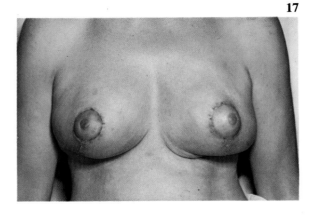

Non-physiological secretion of milk from the breasts is now recognised as a common endocrine problem. A woman may not be aware of the secretion, and expression of the breast is part of the routine endocrine examination of all women with infertility, amenorrhoea, hirsutes, and hypo-thalamic-pituitary disease. The causes of galactorrhoea are discussed in Chapter 1. Brown or blood-stained secretion should alert the clinician to the possibility of a breast tumour. These conditions are not dealt with in this book.

18

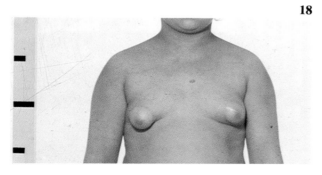

Apparent overgrowth of the areolae is common during puberty (**18**) and gradually recedes as full breast development occurs. Stimulation of the nipple causes contraction of the local musculature and a more normal appearance is restored.

7: Diabetes mellitus

Introduction

Diabetes mellitus is the term given to a syndrome which has as its most prominent feature elevation of the blood glucose with subsequent glycosuria. The elevation of the blood glucose may be asymptomatic, but the glycosuria causes an osmotic diuresis with polyuria, secondary polydipsia and weight loss. The hyperglycaemia of diabetes results from abnormalities of insulin secretion or action, secretion being deficient, delayed or otherwise inappropriate for the prevailing blood glucose level, or its action being affected by circulating antagonists e.g. antibodies or by abnormalities of its tissue receptors.

Classification of diabetes mellitus

Hereditary idiopathic diabetes mellitus (sometimes autoimmune)
Subclinical
a) Prediabetes or potential diabetes where there is no abnormality of carbohydrate metabolism even after steroid administration but the individual is at risk for the future development of the condition.

b) Latent diabetes refers to normal individuals who develop impairment of carbohydrate metabolism in response to stress or steroids.

c) Chemical diabetes refers to patients with glycosuria, hyperglycaemia and impaired carbohydrate tolerance who are asymptomatic.

Overt diabetes
  a) Juvenile onset
  b) Maturity onset

Secondary to pancreatic disease
After acute or chronic pancreatitis
Haemochromatosis
After pancreatectomy
Tumours
After removal of an islet cell tumour (usually transient)

Related to other endocrine syndromes
Cushing's syndrome
Acromegaly
Phaeochromocytoma
Hyperthyroidism
Aldosteronism

Precipitated by drugs
Thiazide diuretics and diazoxide
Corticosteroids
Oral contraceptives

Related to non-endocrine disease
Chronic renal failure
Liver disease

Clinical features of diabetes mellitus

Other than the sequelae of hyperglycaemia – polyuria, polydipsia and weight loss, the clinical features of diabetes mellitus are those of its acute or chronic complications and those of any underlying cause.

Features of pancreatic diseases causing diabetes

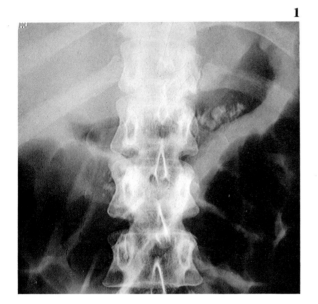

1

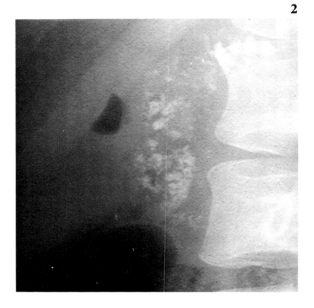

2

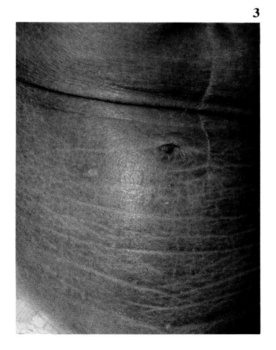

3

Chronic pancreatitis with calcification is a rare cause of diabetes except in certain areas such as Southern India. 1 and 2 show pancreatic calcification.

Haemochromatosis may be recognised by the characteristic bronze skin pigmentation (3) caused by deposits of haemosiderin and melanin, and by the associated hepatosplenomegaly of cirrhosis. Epigastric scars may give a clue to a laparotomy for acute pancreatitis or a pancreatic tumour.

Features of other endocrine diseases causing diabetes

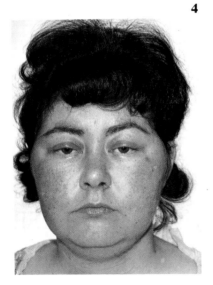

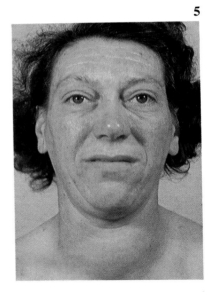

Cushing's syndrome (4) caused by pituitary or adrenal disease or as a result of steroid administration is commonly complicated by diabetes mellitus. Acromegaly (5) is associated with overt or subclinical diabetes in at least one quarter of cases, although this rarely causes any problem in management. Phaeochromocytomas may cause diabetes (note the calcified adrenal tumour (6)).

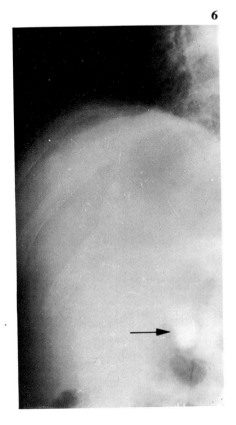

Hyperthyroidism from any cause may precipitate diabetes in pre-diabetic or latent diabetic individuals (7). This condition usually remits with effective antithyroid therapy.

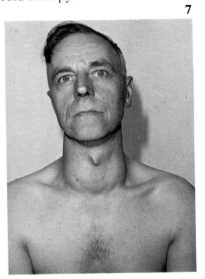

Features of non-endocrine disease causing diabetes

8

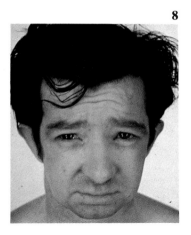

9

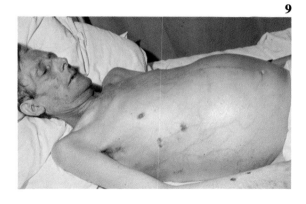

Carbohydrate intolerance is impaired in most patients with chronic renal failure (note the characteristic uraemic appearance (**8**)).

Chronic liver disease of any variety may also be associated with diabetes mellitus. **9** shows a jaundiced, cirrhotic patient with ascites who developed diabetes.

Complications of diabetes mellitus

10

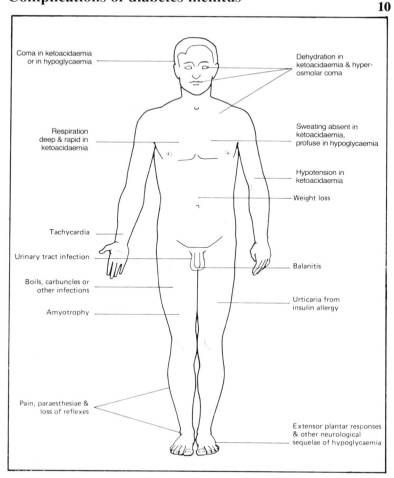

Coma in ketoacidaemia or in hypoglycaemia

Respiration deep & rapid in ketoacidaemia

Tachycardia

Urinary tract infection

Boils, carbuncles or other infections

Amyotrophy

Pain, paraesthesiae & loss of reflexes

Dehydration in ketoacidaemia & hyper-osmolar coma

Sweating absent in ketoacidaemia, profuse in hypoglycaemia

Hypotension in ketoacidaemia

Weight loss

Balanitis

Urticaria from insulin allergy

Extensor plantar responses & other neurological sequelae of hypoglycaemia

Acute complications (10):

Insulin allergy
Hyperlipidaemia
Hypoglycaemia
Diabetic ketoacidaemia (**11** shows the typical dry tongue of a dehydrated diabetic with this condition)
Lactic acidaemia
Hyperosmolar non-ketotic diabetic coma
Acute infections
Acute neuropathy

11

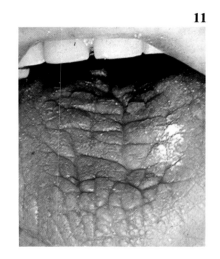

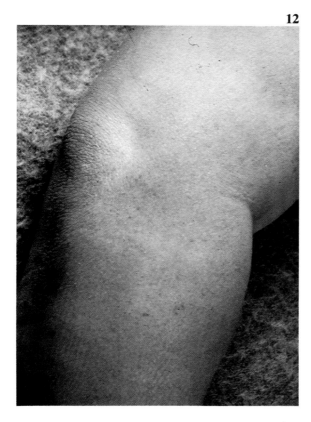

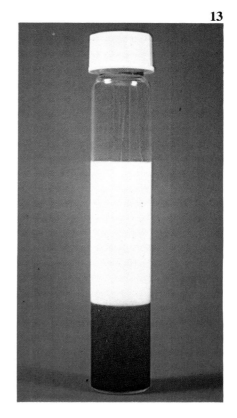

Insulin allergy This condition is uncommon and erythema at the injection site is usually caused by either contaminants or infection. The usual manifestation is urticaria (**12**) but severe anaphylactic shock may occur.

Hyperlipidaemia In diabetic ketoacidosis the serum may appear milky as a result of a gross hyperlipidaemia (**13**); this may be reflected in the fundus by the characteristic lipaemia retinalis (**14**).

Acute infections Acute bacterial infections may affect the skin-boils or carbuncles (**15**) or the urinary tract.

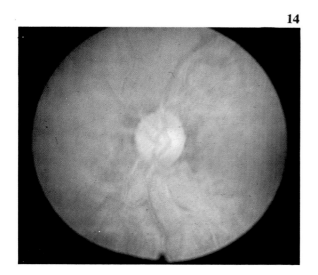

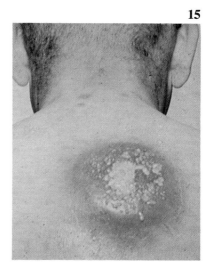

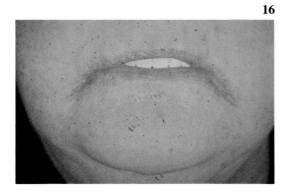

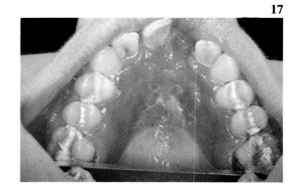

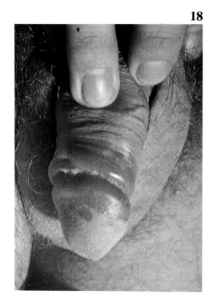

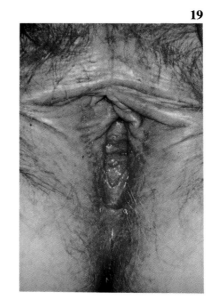

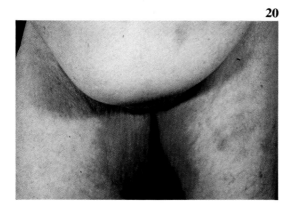

Candida infections of the mouth, such as angular stomatitis (16) or stomatitis (17 shows candidiasis in a denture wearer), or infections of the penis, such as balanitis (18) and of the vagina may occur. Vulvitis in a diabetic is usually caused by candida infection (19) and the infection may spread to the upper inner thighs (20) and skin flexures.

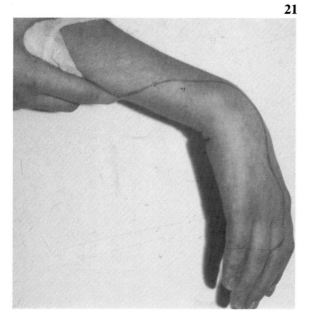

22

Acute neuropathy Acute neuropathy may be seen during or after a period of poor control.

A variety of neuropathic syndromes may be seen affecting motor and sensory nerves in lower and upper limbs, including mononeuritis multiplex. **21** shows wrist drop in a diabetic.

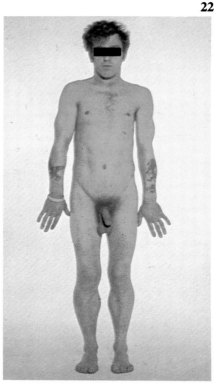

Diabetic amyotrophy is caused by a proximal radiculopathy; muscle wasting affecting the thighs is common (**22** shows wasted thighs which contrast with the well developed calves), and upper motor neurone lesions may also be present.

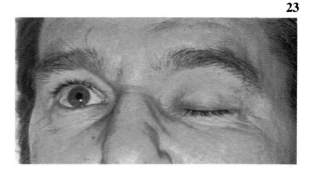

Isolated cranial nerve palsies e.g. of the III nerve (**23**) are probably of vascular origin.

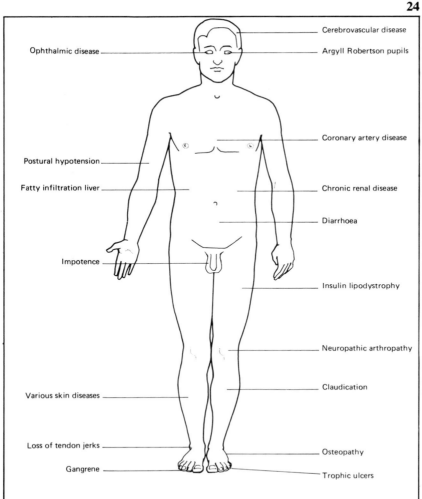

Chronic complications (24)

Insulin lipodystrophy
    Hypertrophy
    Atrophy

Fibrosis at injection sites
Atherosclerosis
Renal disease
Chronic neuropathy
Ophthalmic disease
    Disturbance of visual
    acuity
    Cataracts
    Iridopathy
    Retinopathy

Dermatological disease
    Pyogenic infections (*vide supra*)
    Candidiasis (*vide supra*)
    Pseudoxanthoma nigricans
    Diabetic dermopathy
    Xanthoma diabeticorum
    Necrobiosis lipoidica
    Granuloma annulare

Chronic infections
Diabetic foot disease and osteopathy

Labels on figure:
Cerebrovascular disease
Argyll Robertson pupils
Ophthalmic disease
Coronary artery disease
Postural hypotension
Fatty infiltration liver
Chronic renal disease
Diarrhoea
Impotence
Insulin lipodystrophy
Neuropathic arthropathy
Claudication
Various skin diseases
Loss of tendon jerks
Osteopathy
Gangrene
Trophic ulcers

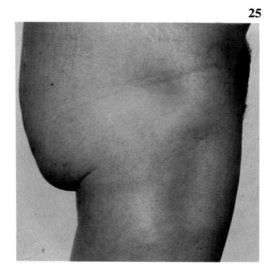

25

Insulin lipodystrophy This occurs at the site of insulin injections. Hypertrophy consists of soft lipomatous swellings caused by an increase in total lipid and hypertrophied fat cells (**25**). The condition is common in those under 20 years of age. Atrophy is caused by loss of fatty tissue (**25**). It may improve spontaneously or after injections of neutral insulin into the affected area.

Fibrosis at injection sites This causes variability in the rate of insulin absorption.

26

27

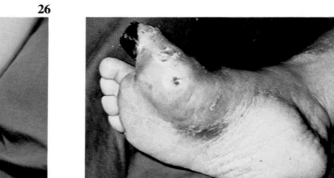

Atherosclerosis This appears earlier and is more extensive in diabetics. It may affect any of the characteristic sites seen in non-diabetics. Limb vessel involvement may lead to intermittent claudication or gangrene (**26**), such lesions being even more prone to infection in the diabetic (**27**).

28

An underlying osteitis may be revealed on X-ray (**28**). Visceral vessel involvement may cause ischaemic heart disease; the frequency of angina pectoris and myocardial infarction is increased in diabetics, or in those with premature cerebrovascular disease. Atherosclerosis may also play a part in some of the other chronic complications of diabetes, namely glomerulosclerosis, retinopathy, and neuropathy. It must be distinguished from the characteristic vascular lesion in diabetes – the microangiopathy which is mainly responsible for the nephropathy, retinopathy and neuropathy as well as for some of the skin lesions. The specific basement membrane thickening of diabetic microangiopathy may affect all arterioles, venules, and capillaries to a greater or lesser extent.

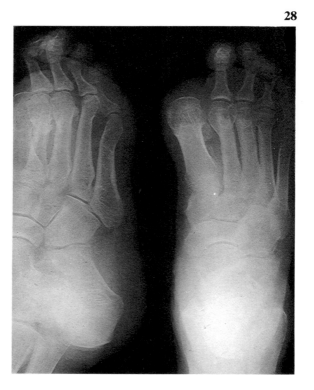

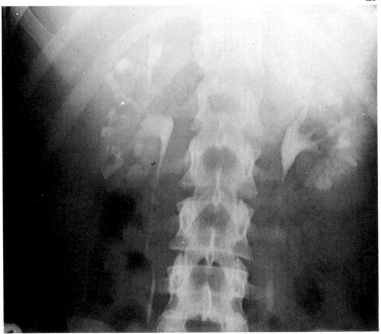

Renal disease This condition may be non-specific, for example, due to pyelonephritis (**29** is a pyelogram showing the loss of renal cortex and clubbing of the calyces), nephrosclerosis or hypertension or may be due to a specific diabetic glomerulosclerosis, the Kimmelstiel–Wilson syndrome. This may produce typical clinical features of the nephrotic syndrome with facial and generalised oedema. **30** shows gross pitting oedema in a patient with the nephrotic syndrome.

30

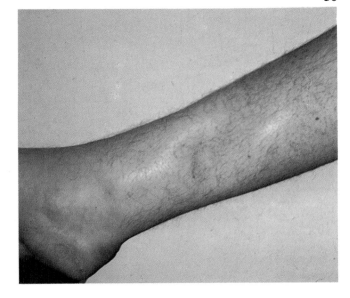

Chronic neuropathy This condition probably results from a combination of atherosclerosis and microangiopathy. It may comprise the following:

a) Sensory nerve involvement which can lead to trophic ulceration (**31**) and neuropathic arthropathy: a Charcot joint (**32** and **33**).

b) Motor nerve involvement causes muscle weakness and wasting.

c) Autonomic nerve involvement causes pupillary changes (Argyll–Robertson pupils), dependent oedema, reduced sweating, bowel, bladder and sphincter disturbances, reduced potency, and postural hypotension.

31

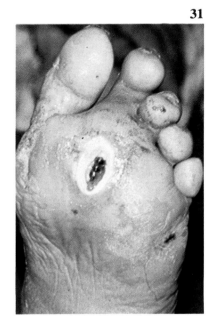

32

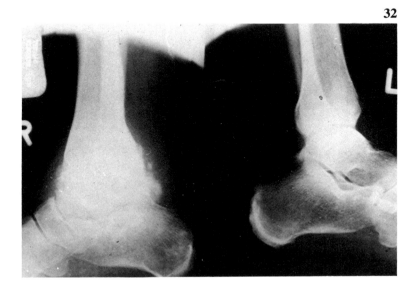

33

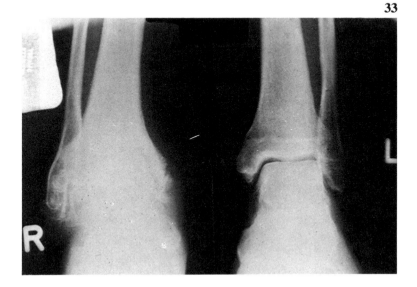

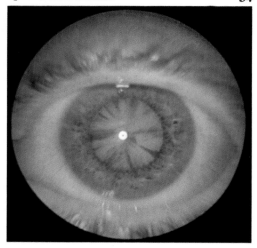

Disturbances of visual acuity These disturbances are common in young diabetics, with widely fluctuating blood sugar levels being largely caused by differences in osmotic pressure between the lens and the extracellular fluid.

Cataracts (34) These are specifically caused by diabetes; they are rare but can occur in young patients when they are usually bilateral, with a snowflake appearance in the subcapsular region of the lens. Senile cataracts occur more frequently and at an earlier age in diabetics.

Iridopathy This condition is seen in some poorly-treated younger diabetics where glycogen is deposited in the pigment epithelium of the posterior surface of the iris. Later a meshwork of new blood vessels develops over the anterior surface of the iris eventually encircling the pupil. Glaucoma is the final result of this process.

35

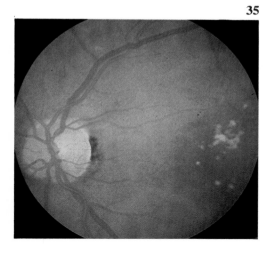

36

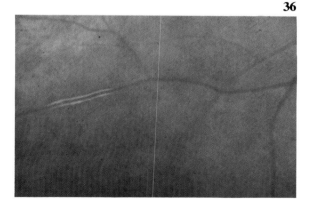

Retinopathy This may be non-specific resulting from hypertensive or atherosclerotic changes or may be specific resulting from diabetic micro-angiopathy.

The lesions of diabetic retinopathy are as follows:

a) Venous changes consist initially of generalised dilatation of veins (35 shows venous dilatation and also microaneurysms within circinate hard exudates); later beading, tortuosity, varicosities, and sheathing (36) may precede the development of microaneurysms.

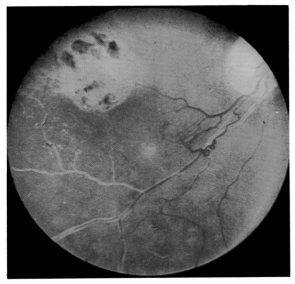

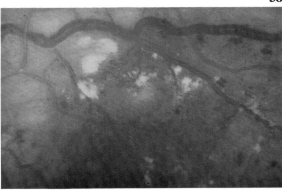

c) Microaneurysms are the characteristic feature of diabetic retinopathy resembling punctate haemorrhages of variable size scattered through the posterior pole and in the macular region. **38** shows microaneurysms, exudates and venous dilatation.

b) Arterial changes consisting of hyalinisation and narrowing of arteries (**37** showing hyalinisation of vessels and also choroidoretinitis) may be partly the result of atherosclerosis.

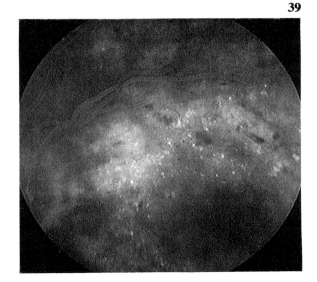

Fluorescence angiograms show up many more than can be seen on routine fundoscopy (**39** and **40**).

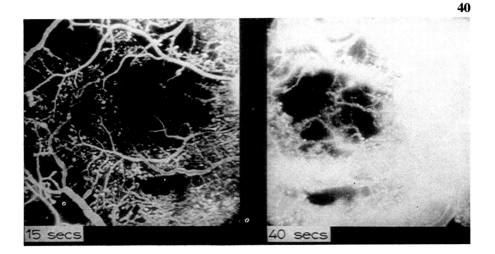

15 secs   40 secs

41

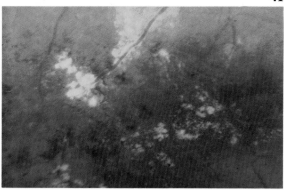

42

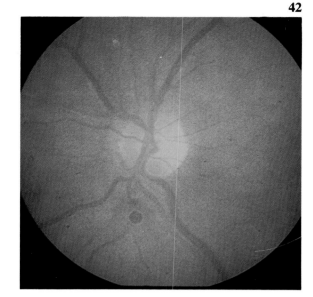

43

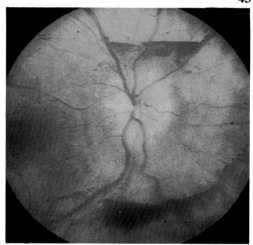

d) Haemorrhages are round and red and are larger than microaneurysms. **41** shows haemorrhages and exudates. **42** shows a pre-retinal smudge haemorrhage on the retinal surface below the disc. **43** shows two large flat-topped subhyaloid haemorrhages. Fluorescein angiography can be used to demonstrate that such haemorrhages are pre-retinal, in front of the retinal vessels, because they mask the intravascular fluorescein (**44**).

44

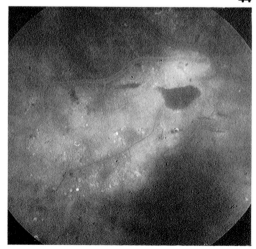

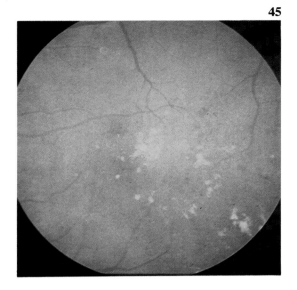

45

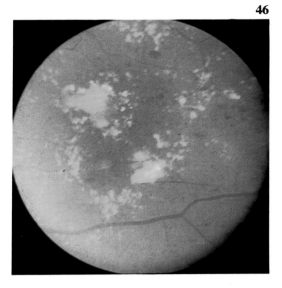

46

e) Exudates are usually hard and white or yellowish in colour. **45** shows circinate retinopathy with hard exudates located in the area of the macula.

46 shows a typical diabetic background retinopathy with larger exudates and microaneurysms.

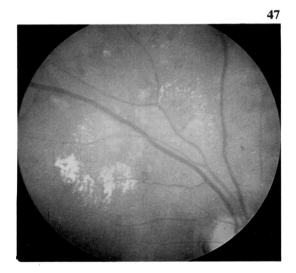

47

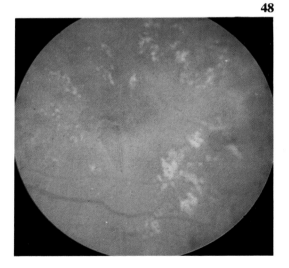

48

f) Cottonwool spots are retinal infarcts resulting from arterial occlusion (**47**) and are a bad prognostic sign. They are contrasted here with hard exudates in two circinate patches. Note the relative independence of the two processes with random scattering of the cottonwool spots over the circinate pattern.

g) Macular disease is an important cause of blindness. Exudates, microaneurysms or haemorrhages may contribute to macular disease, but the major cause of visual impairment is macular oedema. **48** shows early microcystic macular oedema which was confirmed by fluorescein angiography.

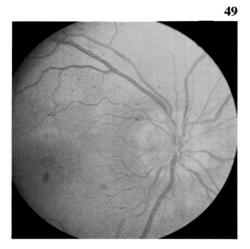

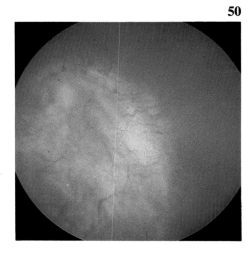

h) Vitreous haemorrhages occur from new vessels as part of the proliferative retinopathy of diabetes. They appear as a haze or as a red or black reflex on fundoscopy (**49**). Later fibrosis may lead to retinal detachment. **50** shows traction of the retina into the vitreous after organisation of a vitreous haemorrhage and contraction of the resultant connective tissue. Vitreous haemorrhages absorb and may form vitreous floaters.

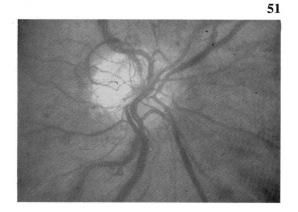

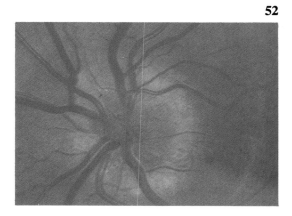

i) Proliferative retinopathy, the formation of new vessels, is a serious feature of diabetic retinopathy. They may be flat on the disc (**51**), mimic papill-oedema (**52**) extend forward into the vitreous (**53** and **54**) or involve the macula.

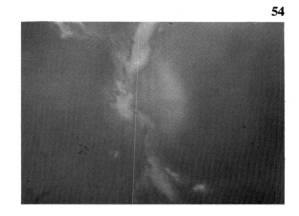

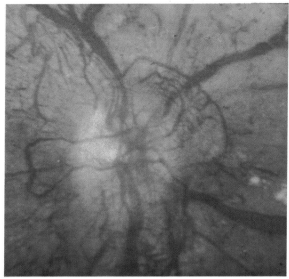

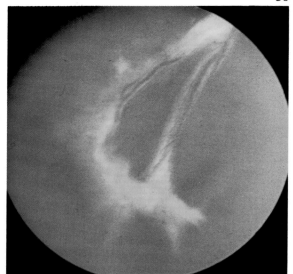

Haemorrhage is frequent (**55**), leading to fibrosis (**56**), distortion of the vitreous and tearing of the retina (*vide supra*).

Classification of diabetic retinopathy

Patients are classified according to the changes present in the more severely affected eye.

Malignant retinopathy includes those with preretinal haemorrhages, new vessel formation or fibrous proliferation, retinal detachment or secondary glaucoma.

Simple retinopathy consists of microaneurysms, retinal haemorrhages and exudates.

Effects of treatment

Photocoagulation produces an iatrogenic choroidoretinitis with characteristic appearance.

Clofibrate may reduce the number of exudates.

Hypophysectomy by surgery or yttrium-90 can sometimes cause dramatic improvement in retinopathy.

Dermatological disease

Pyogenic infections These conditions are common: boils, furunculosis (**57**) and carbuncles from staphylococcal infection are a feature of poorly controlled diabetes.

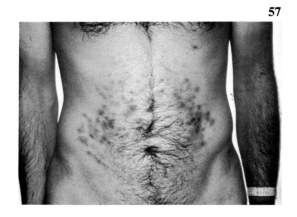

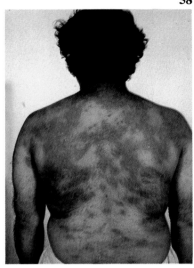

57

58

Candidiasis This is common (see also 'acute complications' page 136), affecting the vulva, perineum and areas of intertrigo.

Pseudoxanthoma nigricans This condition is seen particularly in obese diabetics. The dusky, pigmented, hyperkeratotic lesions affect the axillae, groins and skin folds round the neck resembling true acanthosis nigricans (**58**), but in the diabetic they are benign.

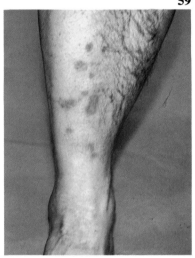

59

Diabetic dermopathy This so-called 'spotted leg' or pigmented pretibial patches (**59**) consists of small pigmented macules or oval pigmented scars in the anterior tibial regions, probably resulting from local trauma.

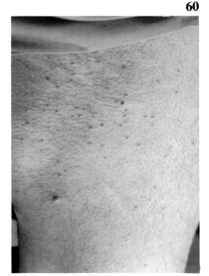

60

Xanthoma diabeticorum **60** shows yellowish papules or nodules occurring on the skin of hyperlipaemia diabetics, which consist of lipid-loaded histiocytes.

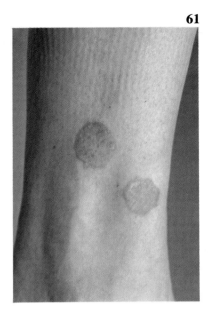
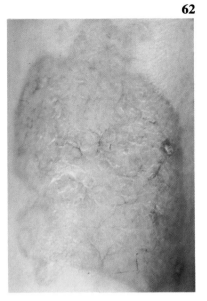
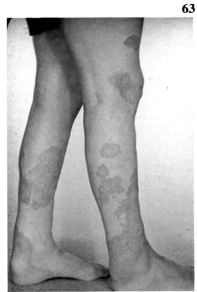

Necrobiosis lipoidica These are asymptomatic lesions involving the leg and are not confined to diabetics. They consist of small papules (**61** and **62**) later enlarging to large plaques resembling localised scleroderma (**63** and **64**), which may ulcerate. Fibrosis and involution may eventually occur.

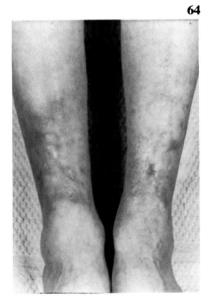

65

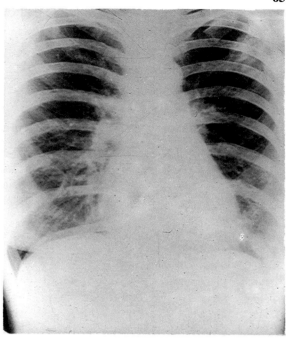

Chronic infections Tuberculosis is common in diabetics. Unexplained weight loss, cough or fever should be an indication for a chest X-ray. **65** shows a tuberculous lesion in the left infraclavicular region in a diabetic. Similarly chronic urinary infections may lead to chronic renal failure.

Diabetic foot disease and osteopathy Foot lesions are common in diabetics. Inspection of the feet is part of the routine diabetic examination. Infections between the toes, paronychia, and chronic ulcers may lead to extensive cellulitis and gangrene (**66**). Atherosclerosis, neuropathy – sensory and autonomic, microangiopathy, infection and general debility may all contribute to the feet lesions of diabetes. The end result of such lesions is amputation.

Radiological changes in the feet are common in diabetes consisting of arterial calcification or osteopathy – diffuse or localised osteoporosis leading to juxta-articular bone defects in the phalanges and metatarsals. Later osteolysis of the bone ends (**67**) and destruction of entire bones may occur.

67

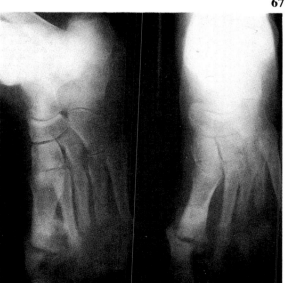

66

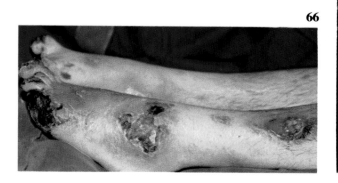

Lipoatrophic diabetes

This rare syndrome consists of non-ketotic insulin resistance, generalised atrophy of adipose tissue, severe hyperlipaemia with subcutaneous xanthomatosis, and hepatosplenomegaly. In one form of the condition, acanthosis nigricans is associated.

DIDMOAD syndrome

In this rare familial syndrome various combinations of diabetes insipidus (DI), diabetes mellitus (DM), optic atrophy (OA) and deafness (D) are seen.

Prader–Willi Syndrome

68

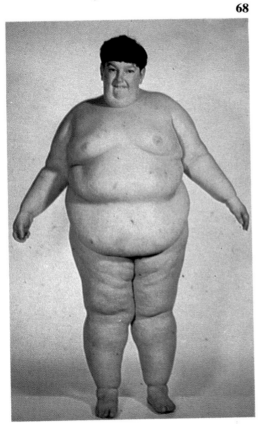

69

70

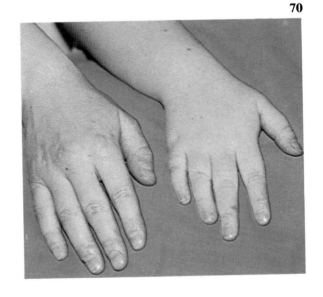

In this rare syndrome diabetes mellitus is a frequent complication of the gross food intake. **68** to **70** show the characteristic features of this syndrome, with marked obesity, small genitalia, and small hands.

8: Pancreatic and gastrointestinal hormones

Pancreatic hormones

The endocrine cells in the pancreas are aggregated in the islets of Langerhans. Specific cells secreting insulin, glucagon and somatostatin have been identified. Clinical syndromes due to tumours of these specific cell types can be recognised.

Insulinomas These tumours cause hypoglycaemia which can present in a wide variety of guises. It is important to differentiate hypoglycaemia caused by an islet cell tumour from factitious hypoglycaemia resulting from self-administration of insulin. Treatment of islet cell tumours with diazoxide can lead to hirsutism (**1**). Islet cell tumours may be associated with other endocrine tumours in the multiple endocrine adenoma MEA Type I syndrome. Table 1 shows the main features of this syndrome (see page 153).

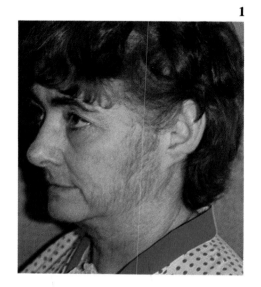

The MEA I syndrome is familial with inheritance on a mendelian dominant basis; patients and their first-degree relatives with one of the diseases shown in Table 1 should be screened for other diseases in the group. Such screening should consist of a clinical examination, skull X-ray, fasting serum calcium and blood glucose estimations. Pituitary, parathyroid and insulin-secreting islet cell adenomas are the commonest cause of disease in the MEA I syndrome.

The MEA II syndrome by contrast is also familial but dominantly inherited. The major features of this syndrome are shown in Table 2 (see page 153).

It should be stressed that there is no overlap either in a patient or her family for the MEA I and II syndromes.

Table 1 MEA I syndrome

Gland	Hormones	Disease
Pituitary	Growth hormone	Acromegaly
	Prolactin	Amenorrhoea, galactorrhoea, impotence
	Corticotrophin	Cushing's disease
	Non-secretory	Hypopituitarism
Parathyroid	Parathormone	Hyperparathyroidism
Thyroid	Thyroid hormones	Subclinical toxic adenoma or toxic nodule
	Non-secretory	Thyroid nodule
Adrenal cortex	Adrenal androgens	Hirsutism, amenorrhoea
	Cortisol	Cushing's syndrome
Pancreas	Insulin	Hypoglycaemia
	Glucagon	Skin rash, glossitis, diabetes
	Gastrin	Zollinger–Ellison syndrome

Table 2 MEA II syndrome

Gland	Hormones	Disease
Thyroid (parafollicular cells)	Calcitonin	Medullary carcinoma of thyroid
Parathyroid	Parathormone	Hyperparathyroidism
Adrenal medulla	Adrenaline, noradrenaline, dopamine	Phaeochromocytoma

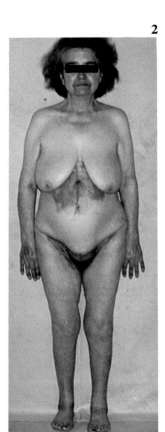

2

Glucagonomas These tumours of the pancreas present with characteristic clinical features. A skin rash is often widespread; lesions, beginning as erythematous areas, become raised with superficial central blistering and rupture to leave crusts or, in areas exposed to friction, weeping (**2** to **6**). The lesions tend to heal in the centre while the edges spread with a red crusting well-defined margin and an annular outline. Healing is associated with increased pigmentation. Circumoral crusting and

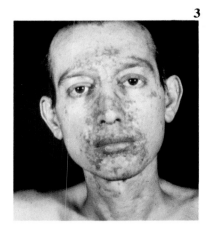

3

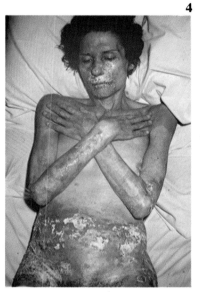

4

painful glossitis are common. The patients also lose weight and are usually diabetic.

Somatostatinomas of the pancreas have been described in two patients.

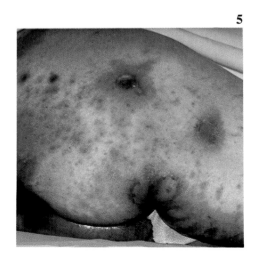

5

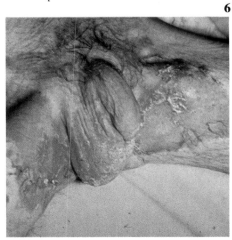

6

Gut hormones

The gut has the largest number of endocrine cells in the body; they are scattered throughout the mucosa as single cells. The aminoacid sequences of six peptides derived from the gut endocrine cells are called: gastrin, secretin, cholecystokinin (CCK), gastric inhibitory peptide (GIP), vaso-active intestinal peptide (VIP), and motilin.

Zollinger – Ellison syndrome

Clinical syndromes are known to result from gut tumours secreting gastrin and VIP. The Zollinger–Ellison syndrome consists of intractable peptic ulceration and gastric hypersecretion resulting from a gastrin-secreting tumour of the pancreas or more rarely the duodenum. On radiology the gastric and duodenal folds are usually coarse (**7** shows a large gastric ulcer with radiating mucosal folds), and there may be duodenal dilatation. The ZE syndrome is also associated with the MEA Type I syndrome.

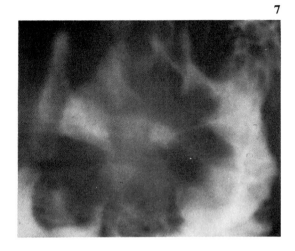

7

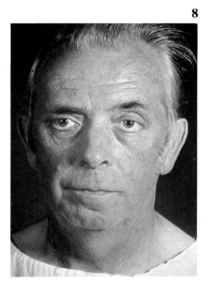

8

Verner – Morrison syndrome

The Verner–Morrison syndrome consists of chronic, profuse, watery diarrhoea which leads to dehydration and hypokalaemia, accompanied by hypoglycaemia, hypochlorhydria, and attacks of flushing (**8**). The pancreatic tumours in these patients contain large amounts of vasoactive intestinal peptide (VIP) and plasma levels of this hormone are elevated. The tumour can sometimes be demonstrated by angiography. **9** shows an angiogram of a pancreatic VIPOMA.

9

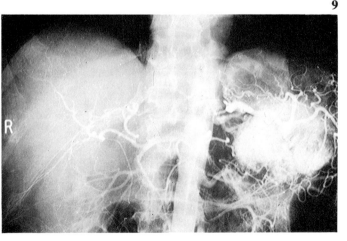

9: Parathyroids

Introduction

The parathyroid glands secrete parathyroid hormone which is concerned with maintaining a normal plasma calcium level. Hypocalcaemia is the most potent stimulus to parathormone secretion; the reciprocal relationship which exists between plasma calcium and parathormone levels results from this normal feedback mechanism.

Clinical features of parathyroid disease

Diseases of the parathyroid glands may present as either hyperparathyroidism or hypoparathyroidism and are grouped as follows:

Hyperparathyroidism
   Primary
   Secondary
   Tertiary

Hypoparathyroidism
   Neonatal
   Postsurgical
   Idiopathic: failure of parathormone secretion
           failure of parathormone action
           (pseudohypoparathyroidism)

1

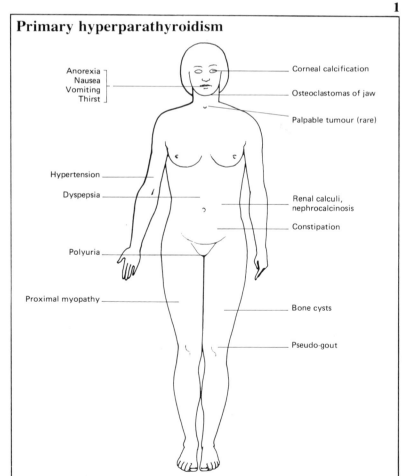

Primary hyperparathyroidism

Anorexia
Nausea
Vomiting
Thirst

Hypertension

Dyspepsia

Polyuria

Proximal myopathy

Corneal calcification

Osteoclastomas of jaw

Palpable tumour (rare)

Renal calculi, nephrocalcinosis

Constipation

Bone cysts

Pseudo-gout

The clinical features of hyperparathyroidism are shown in **1**. Primary hyperparathyroidism may result from the presence of one or more tumours of the parathyroid glands, from hyperplasia of all four glands or rarely from a parathyroid carcinoma.

Presenting features of hyperparathyroidism

Renal disorders Nephrocalcinosis (2) and renal stone formation (3) are common complications of hyperparathyroidism. Because the stones contain calcium they are radio-opaque.

2

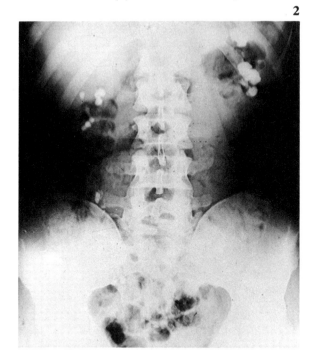

3

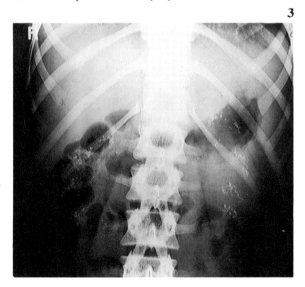

Osteitis fibrosa This causes general aches and pains; sometimes severe bone pain, tenderness and even fractures and deformities can be experienced.

The characteristic radiological signs are subperiosteal erosions of the phalanges and terminal digital tufts (4). Bone cysts may be solitary (5) or multiple (6).

4

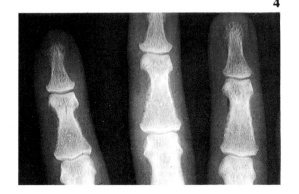

5

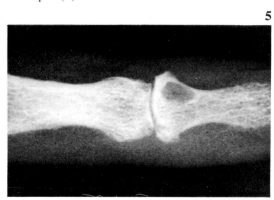

6

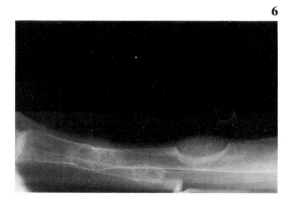

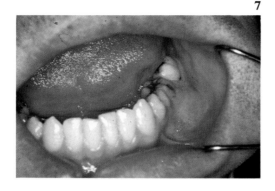

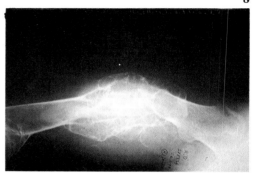

Cysts or osteoclastomas of the jaw (**7**) or a long-bone (**8**) may be presenting features.

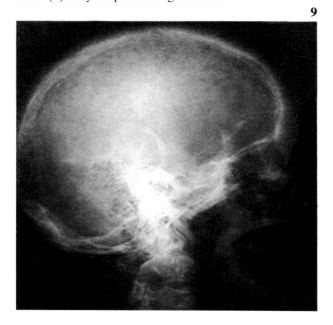

The skull may show a granular or mottled appearance like ground glass and sometimes cystic areas are apparent (**9**).

Loss of the lamina dura may be seen in X-rays of the jaw. **10** shows normal dura around the teeth and its loss in hyperparathyroidism (**11**).

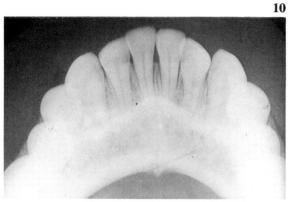

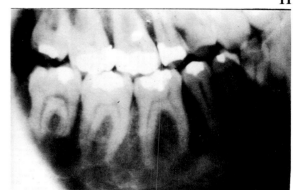

Gastrointestinal symptoms Epigastric pain, with or without peptic ulceration is common. Some patients develop severe constipation, probably as a result of hypercalcaemia. Acute, subacute or chronic pancreatitis may be associated with pancreatic calculi (**12**).

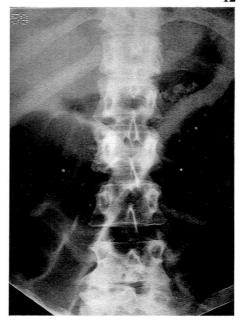

Hypercalcaemia Hypercalcaemia may be responsible for polyuria and polydipsia and for the symptoms of lassitude, nausea or vomiting, muscle weakness, and depression.

Ectopic calcification may be visible in the lateral margins of the cornea (**13**), unlike arcus which first develops at the upper and lower limbi of the cornea and eventually becomes circumferential (**14**).

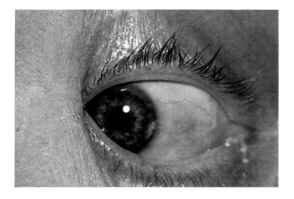

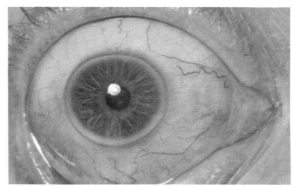

Calcification in joint cartilages is found in some cases. **15** and **16** show chondrocalcinosis in the knee. Calcification may be complicated by pseudo-gout, which particularly affects the shoulders and knees.

15   **16**

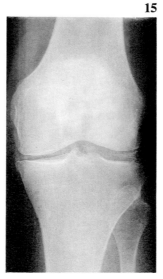

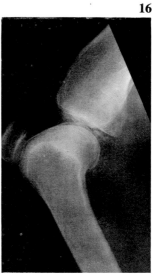

Associated endocrine diseases Hyperparathyroidism may occur in association with other endocrine diseases as part of a pluriglandular syndrome. Multiple endocrine adenoma syndrome I (MEA-I) may consist of a pituitary tumour (acromegaly, Cushing's disease, hyperprolactinaemia or a non-secretory tumour), pancreatic tumour (insulin, gastrin or glucagon-secreting), or adrenal tumour (cortisol or androgen secreting). The MEA-II syndrome consists of medullary carcinoma of the thyroid associated with hyperparathyroidism and phaeochromocytoma.

Differential diagnosis of primary hyperpara-thyroidism

Hypercalcaemia This condition in hyperpara-thyroidism is accompanied by hypophosphataemia, sometimes hyperchloraemia and by an elevated alkaline phosphatase if there are bone lesions. Other important causes of hypercalcaemia include the following:

17 **18**

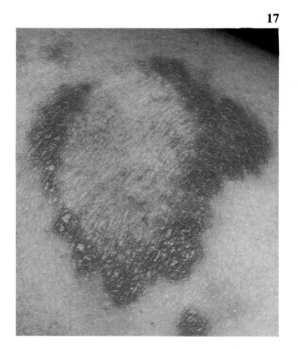 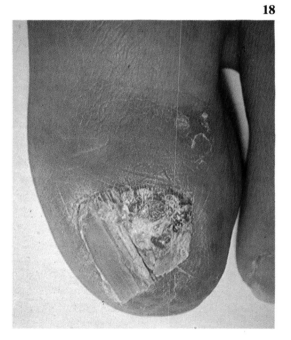

Sarcoidosis – where lupus-like skin infiltration (**17**) nail changes (**18**) and cystic bone lesions (**19**, see next page) may be present.

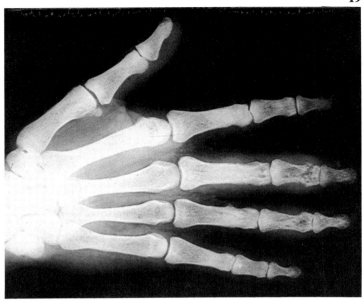

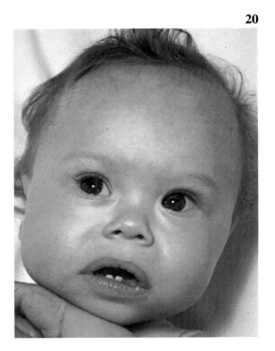

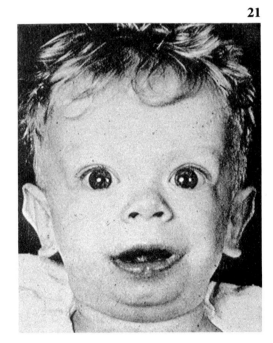

Vitamin D intoxication or sensitivity – the latter being the cause of the 'idiopathic hypercalcaemia of infancy' when the child has a typical elfin appearance (**20** and **21**).

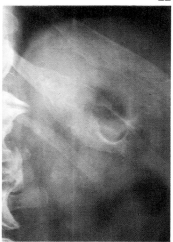

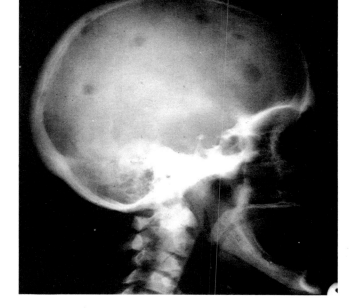

Bone diseases – including oesteolytic secondary deposits (**22**), multiple myeloma (**23**) and Paget's disease (**24** and **25**) and rarely osteoporosis after immobilisation (**26**). The clinical and radiological features of these bone diseases may sometimes be mistaken for hyperparathyroidism.

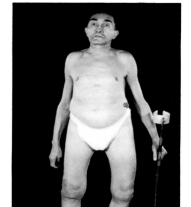

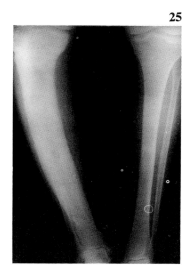

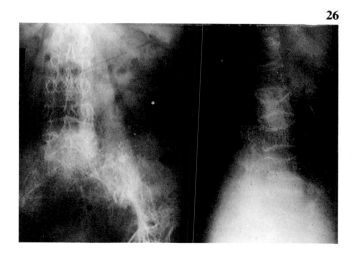

Diagnosis of primary hyperparathyroidism Elevation of the plasma calcium remains the prime diagnostic criterion of hyperparathyroidism. Parathormone levels are not always elevated in current radioimmunoassays, but readily detectable circulating parathormone in the presence of hypercalcaemia lends support to the diagnosis.

Secondary hyperparathyroidism

Secondary hyperparathyroidism is defined as a condition when more parathyroid hormone is manufactured than is normal but where this hormone is needed for some compensatory process. It is common in chronic renal failure. **27** shows an X-ray of secondary hyperparathyroidism in chronic renal failure. Clinical features of the renal failure are usually apparent. **28** shows a patient with the typical uraemic appearance. Osteosclerosis is also seen in some patients with chronic renal failure (**29** to **31**).

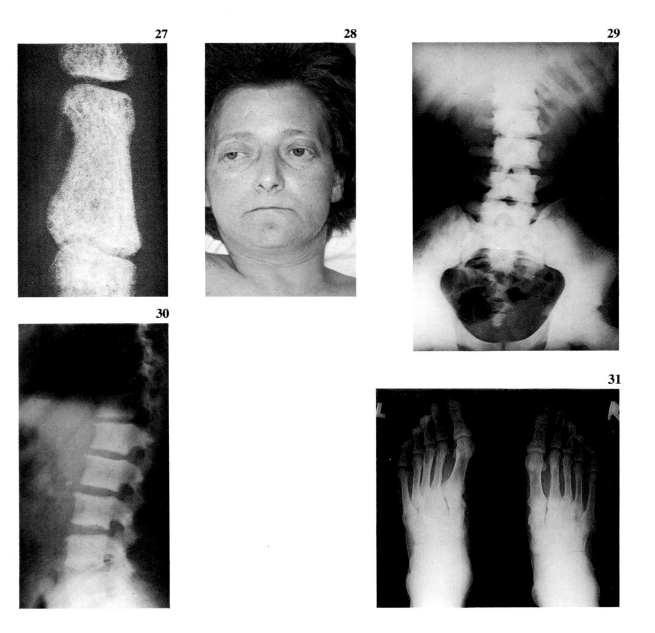

27

28

29

30

31

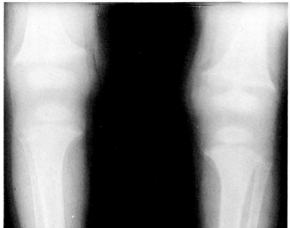

32

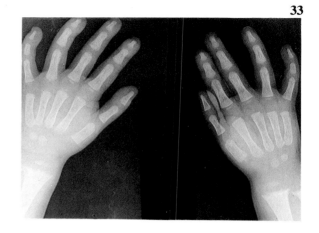

33

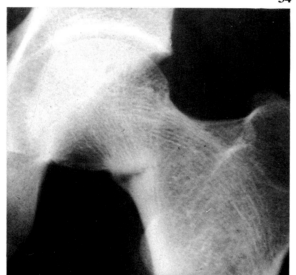

34

Secondary hyperparathyroidism is commonly associated with Vitamin D deficiency in rickets and osteomalacia. **32** and **33** show X-rays of typical bone changes in rickets. **34** and **35** show Looser's zones in the femoral neck and scapula in osteomalacia. Vitamin D deficiency may cause proximal muscle weakness (**36**).

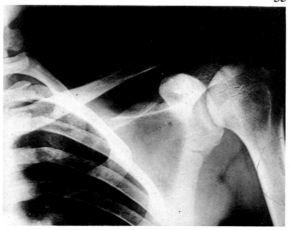

35

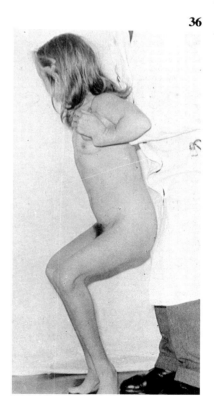

36

Tertiary hyperparathyroidism

37

The term 'tertiary hyperparathyroidism' is used to describe patients who develop parathyroid adenomas causing hypercalcaemia on the background of reactive or secondary parathyroid hyperplasia.

Hypoparathyroidism

37 shows the clinical features of hypoparathyroidism. Hypoparathyroidism results in hypocalcaemia, which causes increased excitability of the neuromuscular junction or the central nervous system.

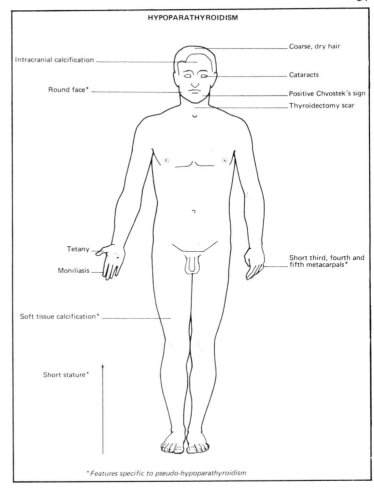

HYPOPARATHYROIDISM

Intracranial calcification
Round face*
Tetany
Moniliasis
Soft tissue calcification*
Short stature*

Coarse, dry hair
Cataracts
Positive Chvostek's sign
Thyroidectomy scar
Short third, fourth and fifth metacarpals*

Features specific to pseudo-hypoparathyroidism

Aetiology of hypoparathyroidism

Neonatal hypoparathyroidism This is a cause of hypocalcaemic convulsions in the children of mothers with hyperparathyroidism, which resolves spontaneously.

Post-surgical hypoparathyroidism This is a dangerous complication of surgery in the neck, usually after partial or total thyroidectomy (**38**). The plasma calcium should be checked in all patients after thyroidectomy; remember that hypocalcaemia could be a possible cause of any non-specific symptoms in a patient who has undergone thyroidectomy.

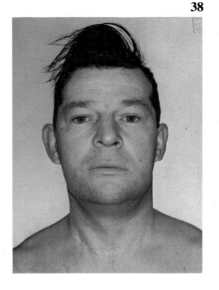

38

Idiopathic hypoparathyroidism This results from failure of parathormone secretion or from failure of its peripheral action.

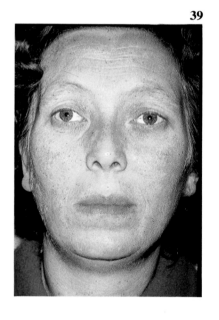

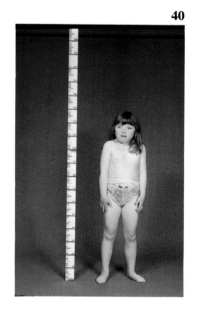

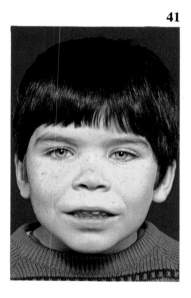

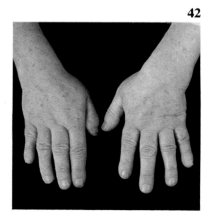

Failure to secrete parathyroid hormone may be familial and is sometimes associated with idiopathic (autoimmune) Addison's disease (**39**). Failure of parathormone action occurs in the syndrome of pseudohypoparathyroidism, a familial condition characterised by mental retardation, short stature (**40**) a characteristic round face (**41**) and shortness of the third, fourth and fifth metacarpals. **42** shows the normal fingers compared with the typical short fingers in **43** and **44**.

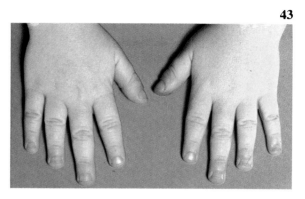

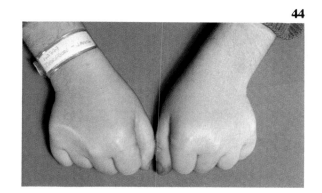

X-rays of the hands (**45**) and feet (**46**) demonstrate the short metacarpals and metatarsals respectively.

The term 'pseudo-pseudohypoparathyroidism' is used to refer to patients with the skeletal abnormalities of pseudohypoparathyroidism without the biochemical disorder.

45

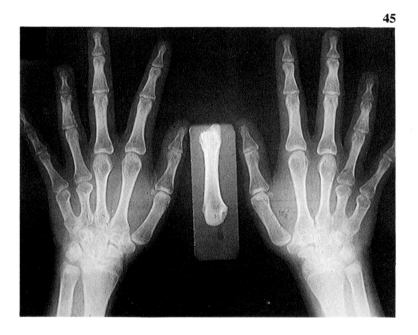

46

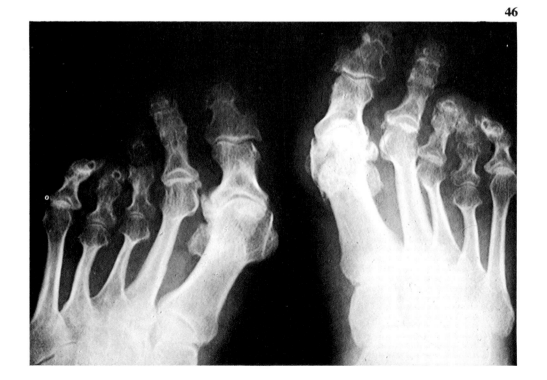

Clinical features of hypoparathyroidism

Tetany This is a complex of symptoms and signs resulting from hypocalcaemia and includes the following:

Paraesthesiae of the hands, feet and circumoral region.

47

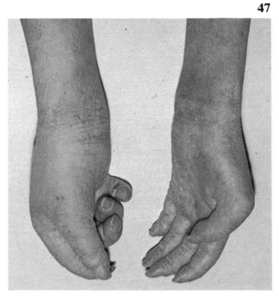

Carpopedal spasm when the fingers take up a characteristic position (**47**). This can be induced in hypocalcaemic patients by occluding the circulation to the arm – Trousseau's sign.

Neuromuscular irritability may be produced by tapping the facial nerve in front of the ear causing twitching of the facial muscles – Chvostek's sign.

49

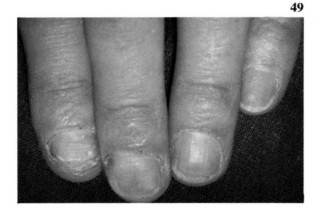

48

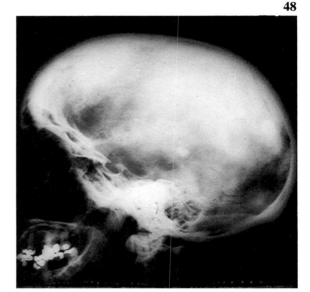

Other features of hypocalcaemia

Epilepsy and mental deterioration may result from hypocalcaemia and psychological disturbances are common.

Intracranial sequelae of hypocalcaemia include raised intracranial pressure and papilloedema and symmetrical, bilateral calcification of the basal ganglia (**48**).

Cataracts may result from long-standing hypocalcaemia of any cause.

Hair and skin lesions The skin and hair may be coarse and dry and the nails brittle and deformed. Moniliasis of the skin and nails (**49**) is often resistant to therapy.

Index

Index